Nancy Clark's
FOOD
GUIDE *for*
MARATHONERS

TIPS FOR EVERYDAY CHAMPIONS

Nancy Clark, MS, RD

Director of Nutrition Services
SportsMedicine Associates
Brookline, MA

Foreword by
John "the Penquin" Bingham

Sports Nutrition Publishers
West Newton, MA

Publisher's Cataloging-in-Publication

Clark, Nancy 1951-
    Nancy Clark's food guide for marathoners: tips for everyday champions/Nancy Clark
    p. cm
    Includes bibliographical references and index.
    LCCN 2002102906
    ISBN 0-9718911-0-9

    1. Runners (Sports)—Nutrition. 2. Marathon running.
    I. Title. II. Title: Food guide for marathoners

TX361.R86C532002   613.2'0247964
                          QBI02-200238

Published in West Newton, MA by Sports Nutrition Publishers,
60 Lindbergh Avenue, Suite 2A, West Newton MA 02465
617-795-0823 sportsnutrition@rcn.com

Book design by Patricia Robinson, Waban, MA parobinson@attbi.com

This book is available at special discounts for bulk purchase. Special editions or book excerpts can also be created to specification. For details, contact the sales manager at Sports Nutrition Publishers.

Printed in the United States of America 10 9 8 7 6 5 4 3 2 1

Photography credits:
Photographs on pages 13, 115 by Bob Fitzgerald, FitzFoto, *New England Runner*
Potographs on pages 19, 21, 79, 95, 96, 103, 105 by Jim Newsom, Joints in Motion
Photographs on pages 47, 50, 57, 122 by Victah Sailer/PhotoRun
Photograph on page 10 by Oleg Shpyrko, Cambridge Sports Union
Photographs on pages 37, 64, 76, 77, 80, 87 by BAA Boston Marathon/FAYFOTO/Boston

The information contained in this book is not intended to serve as a substitute for professional medical advice. The author and publisher specifically disclaim any and all liability arising directly or indirectly from the use of any information contained in this book. A health care professional should be consulted regarding your specific medical and nutritional concerns.

♻ Printed on recycled paper using soy-based ink.

*I dedicate this book to the marathoners
who give of their time and energy to raise money
for important causes and help make the world a better
place. The least I can do is help these everyday champions
enjoy high energy and good health throughout their
marathon experiences by teaching them how to eat effectively.*

CONTENTS

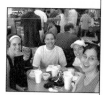

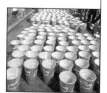

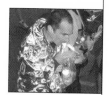

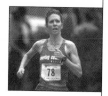

ACKNOWLEDGEMENTS

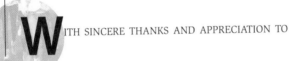

WITH SINCERE THANKS AND APPRECIATION TO

Jenny Hegmann, M.S., R.D., nutrition writer and editor, for her meticulous editing skills.

Patricia Robinson, graphic artist, for producing a delicious-looking book.

Photographers Jim Newsom/Team in Training, Bob Fitzgerald and Michelle LeBrun/New England Runner, Victah Sailer/PhotoRun and the Boston Athletic Association/FayFoto for their contributions.

Recipe contributors Barbara Day, Natalie Updegrove Partridge, Peter Hermann and Gloria Averbusch.

John McGrath, my husband and business partner, for his skillful help with getting this book published.

My clients, many of whom are marathoners, for sharing their experiences. By understanding their nutrition questions and concerns, I am able to better help other marathoners.

The many marathoners in the Joints in Motion and Team in Training marathon training programs who provided guidance for this book.

My children, Mary and John Michael, for their patience with enduring the marathon experience of creating this book.

WHEN I BEGAN MY LIFE AS A MARATHONER, AT 43 YEARS OLD AND 240 pounds, food became my training partner, coach, and competition. But before then, food was a four-letter word. At least it was for me. Actually, food was everything except food. It was love. It was comfort. It was hope. It was recreation. It was a good friend.

I turned to food when I was up, when I was down, and when I was heading from one extreme to the other. Food was my traveling companion, schoolmate, and colleague. It was the first thing I wanted when I woke up and the last thing I thought about before going to sleep.

Like many inexperienced adult-onset marathoners, I transferred my ignorance and obsessions about food to my new life of athletics. I read about what real runners eat and then ate the same way. I bought every magic supplement and tried every new energy bar, gel, and sports drink.

Eventually I learned there's no secret potion that will transform a sedentary, middle-aged man into an Olympian. There's only the slow, steady progress that comes from consistent training fueled by consistent, healthful eating. I learned what to eat by understanding why to eat. I learned about myself, my body, and the food I put into it.

Nancy Clark's Food Guide for Marathoners is perfect for athletes like me. Nancy understands that marathoners come in all sizes, shapes, and in every imaginable combination of talent, desire, and discipline. She understands their struggles with managing time, making meals, and choosing healthy foods in the fast-food American diet.

I had thought that if I wanted to be an athlete, I'd have to eliminate all the foods I enjoyed and learn to like all the foods I'd avoided most of my life. I thought I'd have to give up the joy I found in food. But this wasn't the case. Thanks to Nancy, athletes like me can learn to enjoy food as a fundamental part of training and completing marathons.

Nancy Clark has long been recognized as one who can make complicated, confusing, and often conflicting information about sports nutrition understandable and applicable to athletes of all levels. Whether this is your first week as a marathoner or you're putting the finishing touches on your training diet, Nancy Clark speaks your language. In *Food Guide for Marathoners*, Nancy's considerable skill as a writer and her vast experience as a nutritionist give a much needed common sense perspective on how to fuel easily and effectively for energy, health, and weight management.

Nancy Clark continues to be an enthusiastic cheerleader and preeminent teacher for sensible eating in the sports nutrition community. She'll help you make it to the finish line.

—John Bingham

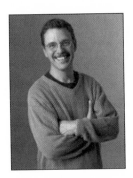

John Bingham has been called the Pied Piper of the 2nd running boom. Through his popular column "The Penguin Chronicles" in Runner's World *magazine and his books* The Courage to Start: A Guide to Running for Your Life *(Simon & Schuster, 1999) and* No Need for Speed: A Beginner's Guide to the Joy of Running *(Rodale Press, 2002), John has helped millions of adult-onset athletes discover the satisfaction of literally changing their life one step at a time.*

Eating Well, Running Well—and Enjoying the Process!

EVERY YEAR, THOUSANDS OF ORDINARY MORTALS TAKE A BIG STEP—actually, that's *millions* of steps—and accept the challenge of training for and completing a marathon. These marathoners may not be Olympians, but they sure are *everyday champions*. This book is designed to help these everyday athletes succeed by teaching them how to fuel their bodies appropriately so they can complete their 26.2-mile challenge—and maybe even have energy to spare!

Nancy Clark's Food Guide for Marathoners: Tips for Everyday Champions will help marathoners of all ages and abilities enjoy fueling themselves well for health, enjoyment (of both food and exercise), and performance.

With the desire to improve personal health and fitness, some marathoners pursue the sport as individuals. Others work as part of a team to raise money for important causes. Teams such as the Leukemia & Lymphoma Society's Team in Training, the Arthritis Foundation's Joints in Motion, the Dana Farber Cancer Center's Marathon Team are just a few of the marathon training teams that raise money to help make the world a healthier, happier place.

If you are a novice marathoner, you may be feeling challenged by the task of how to fuel yourself for such an endeavor. The information provided in *Food Guide for Marathoners* will teach you the tricks to optimizing your sports diet. In this book, I show you how to:

> " *Eat wisely, train smart, and strive to be a little better today than you were yesterday.* "
>
> Jonathan Dietrich, Washington, DC

- manage sweet cravings
- lose weight yet have energy to exercise
- choose the best sports foods before, during, and after your workouts
- carbohydrate-load for a marathon
- enhance your lifelong health with good nutrition

Yes, you can eat well and enjoy good food that helps you to exercise well, even when your life is busy and you have limited time to prepare wholesome meals.

Many of the eating tips in *Nancy Clark's Food Guide for Marathoners* are contributed by novices who wish they had known before their marathon what they know now about how to enhance energy, optimize health, lose weight, and balance good nutrition into a busy lifestyle. Amy Singer of Seattle is once such person. She wrote to me recently:

Having never run at all before June, I completed my first marathon in October. I now love running and eating to run. I'm eager to share what I've learned.

You'll find her helpful tips, plus those of many other marathoners, both novice and experienced, in the following pages.

Eat wisely, walk or run well, enjoy your high energy, and be proud of your success!

Nancy Clark, MS, RD
Director of Nutrition Services
SportsMedicine Associates
830 Boylston Street, Suite 205
Brookline, MA 02467

www.nancyclarkrd.com

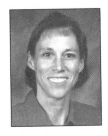

> **❝ Enjoy the means to the end, and always remember to have fun with your training. It's all about learning—from breathing to stretching to eating and drinking on the run (literally) and, yes, learning how to listen to your body (which means rest, too). My first two marathons were awesome; I cherish my finish line photos! ❞**
>
> **Ellen Marie Quinn**
> **Reisterstown, MD**
> **Mentor, Joints in Motion**

Nancy Clark's
FOOD
GUIDE *for*
MARATHONERS

TIPS FOR EVERYDAY CHAMPIONS

CHAPTER 1

Your Daily Diet: What Shape Is It?

WHETHER YOU ARE A WALKER OR A RUNNER, YOUR NUTRITIONAL fitness is as important as your physical fitness. But due to the time constraints that marathon training imposes upon already busy schedules, some runners and walkers fail to plan for meals. Rather, they simply grab whatever is convenient—this may be the same foods day after day, month after month. For example, one of my clients ate spaghetti for breakfast, lunch, and dinner. This repetitive eating kept life simple, minimized decisions, and simplified shopping, but it also created an unbalanced diet and chronic fatigue.

To be nutritionally sound, your diet should include a well-rounded variety of high quality sports foods, such as the cook-free top sports foods listed in the sidebar on page 2. But if you eat a linear diet that lacks variety—for example, bagels, bagels, bagels, or pasta, pasta, pasta—your body will have to chug along on a lackluster intake of vitamins, minerals, and other nutrients.

Take note: You don't have to be a good cook to eat well. Many marathon champs prefer to spend as little time as possible in the kitchen. Yet they still manage to eat well.

If your diet is linear, you might want to reshape it into a well-rounded diet or, better yet, a pyramid. The U.S. Department of Agriculture's

> *I try to live by the 80/20 rule: 80 percent of the time I eat nutritious food; 20 percent of the time I have fun foods as a reward for my hard training. The 20 percent includes chocolate, beer, onion rings, blue cheese, doughnuts, and ice cream.*
>
> Earl Fenstermacher,
> Seattle, WA

The following top sports foods offer mainly cook-free and convenient best bets for people who eat and run.

The best fruits for vitamins A and/or C:
oranges, grapefruit, tangerines, bananas, cantaloupe, strawberries, kiwi

The best vegetables for vitamins A and/or C:
broccoli, spinach, green and red peppers, tomatoes, carrots, sweet potato, winter squash

The easiest sources of calcium for strong bones:
Low-fat milk, yogurt, cheese; calcium-fortified orange juice, soy milk, and tofu

Convenient cook-free proteins for building and protecting muscles:
Deli roast beef, ham, and turkey, tuna, canned salmon, hummus, peanut butter, tofu, cottage cheese

Cook-free grains for carbohydrates and fiber:
High-fiber breakfast cereals (preferably iron-enriched), wholesome breads and bagels, whole-grain crackers

model for healthy eating, the Food Pyramid, reflects the current thinking on nutrition (see the sidebar on page 3). The pyramid shape visually suggests that you should eat lots of grain foods for the foundation of your diet, include generous amounts of fruits and vegetables, and consume lesser amounts of animal proteins and dairy foods. The tiny tip of the pyramid allows for just a sprinkling of sugars and fats.

Not everyone understands the Food Pyramid's messages of *balance, variety,* and *moderation.* Confusion abounds, in particular, regarding the recommended number of servings and how to fit them all into a day's menu:

6–11 servings of grains

2–4 servings of fruits

3–5 servings of vegetables

2–3 servings of milk and dairy foods

2–3 servings of protein-rich foods such as meat and beans.

FOOD PYRAMID   *A Guide to Daily Food Choices*

KEY

■ Fat (naturally occuring and added)

■ Sugars (added)

These symbols show that fat and added sugars come mostly from fats, oils, and sweets, but can be part of or added to foods from the other food groups as well.

Fats, Oils, & Sweets
Use Sparingly

Milk, Yogurt, &
Cheese Group
2-3 Servings

Meat, Poultry, Fish,
Dry Beans, Eggs,
& Nuts Group
2-3 Servings

Vegetable Group
3-5 Servings

Fruit Group
2-4 Servings

Bread, Cereal,
Rice, & Pasta
Group
6-11 Servings

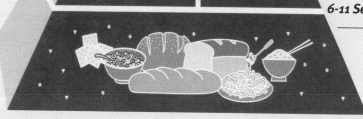

Use the Food Guide Pyramid to help you eat well every day. Start with plenty of Breads, Cereals, Rice, and Pasta; Vegetables; and Fruits. Add two to three servings of foods from the Milk group and two to three servings from the Meat group. Each of these food groups provides some, but not all, of the nutrients you need. No one food group is more (or less) important than another—for good health you need them all. Go easy on fats, oils, and sweets, the foods in the small tip of the Pyramid.

Source: U.S. Department of Agriculture / U.S. Department of Health and Human Services

YOUR DAILY DIET: WHAT SHAPE IS IT?

Although twenty-six servings may sound like several five-course meals, the calories range between 1,600 to 2,800. This is just the right amount of calories for a petite woman on a 1,600 calorie reducing diet or a man who trains for a half-hour per day and requires about 2,800 calories. Your calorie needs likely fall within this range. (See Chapter 13: *Calculating Your Calorie Needs*.)

● BALANCING YOUR DIET

The trick to balancing the recommended servings of foods during your day is to plan to have at least three out of five food groups per meal, and one or two food groups per snack, such as:

	Grain	*Fruit*	*Vegetable*	*Dairy*	*Protein*
Breakfast:	cereal	banana	-----	milk	-----
Lunch:	bread	orange	vegetable soup	-----	peanut butter
Snack:	pretzels	-----	-----	yogurt	-----
Dinner:	spaghetti	-----	tomato sauce broccoli	cheese	ground turkey
Snack:	popcorn	juice	-----	-----	-----

● **CARBOHYDRATES FOR YOUR SPORTS DIET**—By eating according to the Food Pyramid, you'll consume about 55 to 65 percent of your calories from carbohydrates. This is exactly what you need for a high-energy sports diet. These carbohydrates are stored in muscles in the form of glycogen, the energy you need to train hard day after day, and to compete well on race day.

Grain foods are a popular source of carbohydrates for most active people. But even food-loving marathoners may balk at the recommendation to eat six to eleven servings of breads, cereals, and grains *every* day. Some believe they would get fat if they were to eat that much.

But this is not the case. The key to using the Food Pyramid is to understand the definition of "serving." Six to eleven grain servings is only two to four servings per meal (the equivalent of about 150–300 calories), not much for hungry marathoners who require at least 600–900 calories per meal.

Food	Pyramid Serving Size	Marathoner's Portion	Number of Servings
Grains: Recommended Intake—6 to 11 Servings per Day			
Cereal	1 ounce	2–4 ounces (1 big bowl)	2–4
Bread	1 average slice	2 slices in sandwich	2
Bagel	½ small	one large	3–4
Pasta	½ cup cooked	2–3 cups	4–6
Rice	½ cup cooked	1–2 cups	2–4
Fruits: Recommended Intake—2 to 4 Servings per Day			
Orange Juice	6 ounces	12 ounces	2
Apple	1 medium	1 large	2
Banana	1 small	1 large	2
Fruit Cocktail	½ cup	1 cup	2
Vegetables: Recommended Intake—3 to 5 Servings per Day			
Broccoli	1 small stalk	2 large stalks	3–4
Spinach	½ cup	10 ounces (1 box frozen)	3
Salad Bar	1 small bowl	1 large bowl	3–4
Spaghetti Sauce	½ cup	1 cup	2

Fruits and vegetables are also great sources of carbohydrates. But eating the recommended two to four servings per day of fruits and three to five servings per day of vegetables is another story. As one marathoner sheepishly remarked, "I'm lucky if I eat that much in a week." The trick is to eat large portions.

Fruits and vegetables are truly nature's vitamin pills, chock full of vitamin C (to help with healing), beta-carotene (to protect against cancer), fiber (to aid with regular bowel movements), and numerous other vitamins and minerals. The sidebar, *Eat More Veggies!* (page 6), offers suggestions for ways to boost your veggie intake simply.

● **PROTEIN FOR YOUR SPORTS DIET**—Like carbohydrates, protein-rich foods are also an important part of your sports diet. You should eat two to three servings per day. Marathoners tend to

> **"You really don't need to be an expert in deciphering food labels or worrying about what's in a food if you keep shopping simple by sticking to fresh fruits and vegetables and other whole foods."**
>
> Ron Miller, Salt lake City, UT

● EAT MORE VEGGIES!

People who live alone, work long hours, don't cook and/or eat primarily fast foods commonly have vegetable-poor diets. Case in point, Paula, a very busy graduate student, marathoner, and part-time receptionist who confessed, "I know I should eat more vegetables, but I just don't do it. The problem is finding time to buy them and then, staying home long enough to cook and eat them before they go bad. I waste too much money throwing away smelly cauliflower and wilted lettuce."

If you, like Paula, struggle to consume the recommended three to five servings of vegetables per day, the following tips may help you to enhance your nutritional status.

- Eat more of the best, less of the rest. In general, dark green, deep yellow, orange, and red vegetables have far more nutrients than pale ones. Hence, if you dislike pale zucchini, summer squash, and green beans, don't work hard to acquire a taste for them. Instead, put your efforts into having more broccoli, spinach, and winter squash—the richly colored, more nutrient-dense choices.

- Eat colorful salads filled with tomatoes, green peppers, carrots, and dark lettuces and topped with low- or nonfat dressings. Pale salads with white lettuce, cucumbers, onions, celery, and other pale veggies offer little more than crunch. When topped with creamy dressing, this crunch simply becomes a greasy crunch—a far cry from good nutrition. You'd be better off choosing tomato juice, vegetable soups (even canned soups are better than nothing), or a handful of raw baby carrots for a pre-dinner snack.

- Fortify spaghetti sauce with a box of frozen chopped broccoli or green peppers.

either *over-* or *under*consume protein, depending on their health consciousness and lifestyle. Whereas some marathoners fill up on the saturated fat in animal proteins, others bypass these foods in their efforts to eat a low-fat or meat-free diet, but neglect to replace beef with beans. For additional information and guidelines see Chapter 5: *Protein for Marathoners*.

To meet your protein requirement for the day, you should consume not only two to three servings from the protein food group but also the recommended two to three servings of calcium-rich dairy foods such as milk, yogurt and cheese (or other calcium-rich foods, such as calcium-fortified soy milk). Calcium is particularly important for growing teens and

Cook it alongside the spaghetti (in a steamer over the pasta water) or in a covered saucepan with one-half inch of water before you add it to the tomato sauce.

- Choose fast foods with the most veggies:
  - pizza with peppers, mushrooms, and extra tomato sauce
  - Chinese entrées stir-fried with vegetables
  - lunchtime V-8 juice instead of diet soda

- Even over-cooked vegetables are better than no vegetables. If your only option is over-cooked veggies from the cafeteria, eat them. Cooking does destroy some of the vegetable's nutrients, but not all of them. Any vegetable is better than no vegetable!

- Keep frozen vegetables stocked in your freezer, ready and waiting. They are quick and easy to prepare, won't spoil quickly, and have more nutrients than "fresh" vegetables that have been in the store and your refrigerator for a few days. Because cooking (more than freezing) reduces a vegetable's nutritional content:
  - quickly cook vegetables only until tender crisp and use the cooking water as a broth
  - microwave vegetables in a covered dish
  - stir-fry them with very little oil

- When all else fails, eat fruit to help compensate for lack of vegetables. The best alternatives include bananas, oranges, grapefruit, melon, strawberries, and kiwi. These choices are rich in many of the same nutrients found in vegetables.

women who want to optimize bone density. For only 300 calories, even weight-conscious marathoners can not only contribute to their protein intake but also achieve the daily requirement for calcium by consuming:

- 8 oz. of milk or soy milk on breakfast cereal and
- a half-pint (8 oz.) container of skim milk with lunch and
- an 8 oz. cup of yogurt for a snack.

When choosing the recommended two to three daily servings of dairy foods, note that fat-free and low-fat products are preferable for heart-health and calorie control, but you need not suffer with skim milk if you really don't like it. You can always cut back on fat in other parts of your diet. For example, Margie, a first-time

Protein Food	Pyramid Serving Size	Marathoner's Portion	Number of Servings
Tuna	⅓ of 6 oz. can	1 can	3
Chicken	2 ounce drumstick	6 ounce breast	3
Peanut Butter	2 tbsp.	2–4 tbsp.	1–2
Lentil Soup	1 cup	1 bowl	2
Kidney Beans	½ cup	1 cup	1–2

> **I've found that keeping a cooler packed with wholesome foods allows me to graze often and eat the items that fit my dietary requirements. To simplify the process of getting my trough ready, I choose pre-cut fruits and vegetables, dried fruits, nuts, energy bars, yogurt, etc. If I had to work hard at preparing these foods, this plan would quickly fall off my priority list.**
>
> John Correia, San Diego, CA

marathoner, opted for cereal with reduced-fat (2%) milk (five grams of fat per cup), but saved on fat elsewhere in her diet by using fat-free salad dressing and low-fat granola. (For more information on dietary fat, see Chapter 6.)

Runners who prefer a dairy-free diet or are lactose intolerant should take special care to eat adequate amounts of nondairy calcium sources. See the sidebar, *Calcium Equivalents* (page 9), for food suggestions.

● **SWEETS AND TREATS**—Although nutritionists recommend eating a wholesome diet based on grains, fruits, and vegetables from the base of the Food Pyramid, some marathoners eat too many fats, oils, and sweets from the tip. If you have a junk-food diet that topples the tip, you can correct this imbalance by eating more wholesome foods from the base and body of the pyramid *before you get too hungry*. Marathoners who get too hungry tend to choose foods low in nutrients and high in fats and sugar. The simple solution to the junk-food diet is to *prevent* hunger by eating wholesome meals.

The inclusion of fats and sweets in the tip of the pyramid suggests that you need not eat a "perfect diet" (*no* fats, *no* sugar) to have a good diet. Nothing is nutritionally wrong with having a cookie for dessert after having eaten a sandwich, milk, and fruit for lunch. But lots is

The recommended daily calcium intake is:

Age Group	Calcium (mg)
Teens, 9–18 years	1,300
Adults, 19–50 years	1,000
Adults, 51+ years	1,200

Source: Dietary Reference Intakes, National Academy of Science, 1997

The following foods all provide about 300 milligrams of calcium. Two to three choices per day, or one at each meal, will contribute to meeting your calcium needs.

Calcium-rich Foods	Amount
Dairy	
milk, whole or skim	1 cup
yogurt	1 cup
cheese	1½ ounces
cottage cheese	2 cups
frozen yogurt	2 cups
Proteins	
soy milk	1 cup
tofu	8 oz. (½ cake)
salmon, canned with bones	4 ounces
sardines, canned with bones	2½ ounces
almonds	¾ cup
Vegetables	
Broccoli, cooked	3 cups
Collard or turnip greens, cooked	1 cup
Kale or mustard greens, cooked	1½ cups

wrong with eating cookies for lunch and skipping the sandwich. That's when nutrition and performance problems arise.

The key to balancing fats and sugars appropriately in your diet is to abide the following guidelines:

• 10 percent of your calories can appropriately come from refined sugar (about 200–300 calories from sugar per day for most marathoners)

• 25 percent of your calories can appropriately come from fat

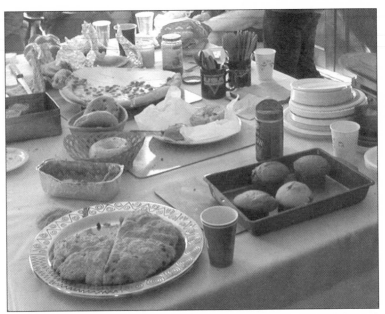

This post-run buffet offers a variety of foods, all of which can be balanced into a well-rounded sports diet. You can enjoy eating treats like scones, pizza, and sweets—just eat them in moderation and choose lower fat foods the rest of the day.

(about 450–750 calories from fat per day, or roughly 50–85 grams of fat per day)

Hence, moderate amounts of chips, salad dressing, jam, and cookies can nourish you with a livable and tasty food plan.

● **WANT SOME HELP SHAPING UP YOUR DIET?**—If you want personalized dietary advice, I recommend that you have a nutrition checkup with a registered dietitian who is interested in sports nutrition. To find a sports nutritionist in your area, call the American Dietetic Association's referral network at (800) 366-1655. Or go to their website at www.eatright.org, enter your zip code into the referral network, and choose from the list of registered dietitians who list "sports nutrition" as a specialty. You'll be glad you did!

Vegetables are the edible parts of plants: the flower (broccoli), berry (pepper), root, bulb, or tuber (carrots, potatoes), stems or shoots (celery, asparagus), or leaves (spinach, lettuce). Vegetables are also excellent sources of "all natural" vitamins that are generally packaged as low fat, carbohydrate-rich sports foods.

Little compares with the nice taste of plain, fresh vegetables cooked until just tender crisp. If you wish to add some seasonings, here are some good combinations:

Basil	Green beans, tomatoes, zucchini
Oregano	Zucchini, mushrooms, tomatoes, onions
Dill	Green beans, carrots, peas, potatoes
Cinnamon	Spinach, winter squash, sweet potatoes
Marjoram	Celery, greens
Nutmeg	Corn, cauliflower, green beans
Thyme	Artichokes, mushrooms, peas, carrots
Parsley	Sprinkled on any vegetable

Saving the Nutrients

To get the most nutrients from your vegetables, handle them properly so they have minimal exposure to the four elements that reduce their nutritional value: air, heat, water, and light.

Problem	Solution
Air	Store fresh vegetables in plastic containers. Cook covered.
Heat	Store fresh vegetables in the refrigerator. Cook only slightly until tender crisp, not mushy. Minimize cooking time to enhance the flavor and nutritional value.
Water	Do not soak vegetables in water. Cook in minimal water, stir-fry, or microwave.
Light	Store in a dark place (inside the fridge!) Cook in a covered pan.

The following tips for cooking vegetables are taken from my *Sports Nutrition Guidebook* (Human Kinetics, 1997).

Basic Steamed Vegetables

1. Wash vegetables thoroughly; prepare and cut into pieces keeping the skin or peel, if appropriate.

2. Put ½ inch water in the bottom of a pan that has a tight cover.

3. Bring the water to a boil. Add the vegetables. Or, put the vegetables in a steamer basket and put this in the saucepan with 1 inch of water.

4. Cover the pan tightly and cook over medium heat until the vegetables are tender crisp, about 3 minutes for spinach, 10 minutes for broccoli, 15 minutes for sliced carrots.

5. Drain the vegetables, reserving the cooking water for soup or sauces, or simply drink it as a broth.

Basic Microwaved Vegetables

Microwave cookery is perfect for vegetables because microwaves cook the veggies quickly and without water, thereby retaining a greater percentage of the nutrients than with conventional methods.

1. Wash the vegetables and cut them into bite-size pieces. Put them in a microwavable container with a cover, or on a plate and then cover with a plastic bag or plastic wrap. If the pieces vary in thickness, arrange them in a ring, with the thicker portions towards the outside of the dish.

   Optional: Sprinkle with herbs (basil, oregano, parsley, garlic powder), soy sauce, or whatever suits your taste.

2. Microwave until tender crisp. The amount of time will vary according to your particular microwave oven and the amount of vegetable you are cooking. Start off with three minutes for a single serving; larger servings take longer. The vegetables will continue cooking after you remove them from the oven, so plan that into your cooking time.

Basic Stir-fried Vegetables

Vegetables stir-fried until tender crisp are very flavorful, colorful, and nutritious, but they do have more fat than if steamed. Be sure to add only a minimal amount of oil (olive, canola, sesame) to the cooking pan. I prefer to use a heavy skillet for stir-frying, rather than a wok—it does a fine job!

Some popular stir-fry combinations include:

- Carrots, broccoli, and mushrooms
- Onions, green peppers, zucchini, and tomatoes
- Chinese cabbage, bok choy, and water chestnuts

1. Wash, drain well (to prevent the water from spattering when the vegetables are added), and cut the vegetables of your choice into bite-sized pieces or ⅛-inch slices. Whenever possible, slice vegetables diagonally to increase the surface area; this allows for faster cooking. Try to make the pieces uniform so they will cook evenly.

2. Heat the skillet or wok over high heat. Add 1 to 3 teaspoons of oil, just enough to coat the bottom of the pan. Optional: Add a slice of ginger root or some minced garlic, stir-frying for one minute to add flavor.

3. Add the vegetables that take longest to cook (carrots, cauliflower, broccoli); a few minutes later add the remaining ones (mushrooms, bean sprouts, cabbage, spinach). Constantly lift and turn the vegetables to coat them with oil.

4. Add a little bit of water (¼ to ½ cup), then cover and steam the vegetables for 2 to 5 minutes. Adjust the heat to prevent scorching.

5. Don't overcrowd the pan. Cook small batches at a time.

6. Optional add-ins: soy sauce, stir-fried beef, chicken, tofu, rice, or noodles.

7. To thicken the juices, stir in a mixture of 2 teaspoons cornstarch diluted into 1 tablespoon water. Add more water or broth if this makes the sauce too thick.

   Optional: Garnish with toasted sesame seeds, mandarin orange sections, or pineapple chunks.

Basic Baked Vegetables

If you are baking chicken, potatoes, or a casserole, you might as well make good use of the oven and bake the vegetables too. Some popular suggestions include:

- Eggplant halves sprinkled with garlic powder
- Zucchini with onions and oregano
- Carrots with ginger
- Sliced sweet potato with apple

1. Put the vegetables (seasoned as desired) in a covered baking dish with a small amount of water, or wrap them in foil.

2. Bake at 350 degrees for 20 to 30 minutes (depending on the size of the chunks) until tender crisp. Caution: With foil-wrapped vegetables, be careful when opening the foil. The escaping steam might burn you.

When you are older, will you be happily enjoying an active lifestyle, as does this eighty year old woman? Perhaps, if you routinely eat meals abundant with fruits, vegetables, and whole grains.

Louise Rosetti, Saugus, MA

CHAPTER 2

Breakfast: The Meal of Champions

GOOD NUTRITION FOR MARATHONERS STARTS AT BREAKFAST. THIS IS the most important meal of the day because it sets the stage for healthful eating. Breakfast eaters tend to eat a more nutritious diet, choose foods lower in fat, have lower blood cholesterol levels, and enjoy success with weight control. They are mentally alert and have more energy to exercise. If you have at least 600 calories in your breakfast budget, you might as well enjoy them so you'll have the energy to spend during your busy day.

If breakfast is so great for us, then why do so many marathoners skip it? They have lots of excuses. But for every excuse to skip breakfast there is an even better reason not to.

I don't have time: If you have no time for breakfast, keep in mind that you can always make time to do what you want to do. Lack of *priority* is the real problem, not lack of time.

Breakfast need not be an elaborate occasion. You can quickly prepare a simple breakfast to eat on the run:

- a baggie filled with raisins and dry cereal
- a pita pocket with a slice or two of low-fat cheese
- a frozen waffle popped into the toaster, then eaten plain, with honey, or with peanut butter

> **Breakfast is not my favorite meal of the day, but I soon learned it was essential to my overall endurance. My training sessions and times were markedly worse when I skipped breakfast. A bagel or cereal in the morning works wonders for me!**
>
> Shelley Smith,
> Highlands Ranch, CO

● NONTRADITIONAL BREAKFASTS

Not everyone likes cereal for breakfast, nor do they want to cook eggs or pancakes. If you are stumped by what to eat for breakfast, choose a food that you enjoy. After all, you'll be more likely to eat breakfast if it tastes good. Remember that any food—even frozen yogurt—is better than nothing.

How about:

- leftover pizza
- leftover Chinese food
- mug of tomato soup
- potato zapped in the microwave while you take your shower
- tuna sandwich
- peanut butter and crackers

- a glass of milk, then a banana while walking to the bus or train
- a travel mug filled with low-fat milk or juice (there will always be coffee at the office), a bagel or bran muffin, and a banana during the morning commute

The key to breakfast on the run is to *plan ahead*. Prepare your breakfast the night before so that you can simply grab it and go during the morning rush. For example, on the weekends, you might want to make banana bread (see my favorite recipe, page 20) or buy a dozen bagels. Pre-slice the loaf and the bagels, wrap the slices in individual plastic bags, and put them in the freezer. Take one or two out of the freezer at night so breakfast will be ready and waiting in the morning.

Breakfast interferes with my training schedule: If you are an early morning runner or walker (5:00–7:00 A.M.), you will likely exercise better and avoid an energy crash if you put just a little gas in your tank before leaving (assuming your stomach can tolerate food, of course). Coffee with extra milk, a swig of juice, a chunk of bagel, or piece of bread are popular choices that can get your blood sugar on the upswing, contribute to greater stamina, and help you feel more awake. If you prefer to abstain, at least have a hefty bedtime snack the night before. (Chapter 8: *Fueling Before You Exercise* explains in greater detail the importance of morning food.)

BREAKFAST: THE MEAL OF CHAMPIONS

Needless to say, all cereals are not created equal. Some offer more nutritional value than others. Here are four tips to help you make the best choices.

1. *Choose iron-enriched cereals with at least 25 percent of the Daily Value for iron to help prevent anemia.*

   Note, however, the iron in breakfast cereals is poorly absorbed compared to the iron in lean red meats. But you can enhance iron absorption by drinking a glass of orange juice or enjoying another source of vitamin C (such as grapefruit, cantaloupe, strawberries, or kiwi) along with the cereal. *Any* iron is better than no iron.

   If you tend to eat "all-natural" types of cereals, such as granola and shredded wheat, be aware that these types have "no additives," hence no added iron. You might want to mix and match all-natural brands with iron-enriched brands (or make the effort to eat iron-rich foods at other meals).

2. *Choose fiber-rich bran cereals with more than 5 gram of fiber per serving.*

   Fiber not only helps prevent constipation but also is a protective nutrient that may reduce your risk of colon cancer and heart disease. Bran cereals are the best sources of fiber, more so than even fruits and vegetables. Choose from All-Bran, 40% Bran Flakes, Raisin Bran, Fruit & Fibre, Corn Bran, Oat Bran, or any of the numerous cereals with "bran" in the name. You can also sprinkle raw bran on low-fiber corn flakes, shredded wheat, and muesli to boost their fiber value.

Breakfast is equally important if you exercise at mid-day or in the afternoon. You need to fuel up in order to do a quality workout that afternoon. Breakfast is essential if you are doing double workouts. Because your muscles are hungriest for carbohydrates within the first two hours after hard exercise, a quick and easy recovery breakfast will set the stage for a strong second workout.

I sometimes hear marathoners express the concern that eating breakfast interferes with their upcoming workout; that the food will sit heavily in the stomach or "talk back." This is unlikely. A low-fat meal at 7:00 to 8:00 A.M. (such as cereal and low-fat milk) should be well digested by noontime. Try it; you'll probably see a positive difference in your energy level.

Note: If you have very loose bowels, you may want to forego bran cereals. The extra fiber may aggravate the situation.

3. *Choose cereals with whole grains listed among the first ingredients.*

Whole wheat, brown rice, corn, and oats are among the grains popularly eaten in breakfast cereals. These should be listed first in the ingredients.

Some runners overlook a cereal's grain content and notice only the sugar or salt content. Remember:

- Salt (sodium) in cereal is a concern if you have high blood pressure. Most runners have low blood pressure and will suffer no health consequences from choosing cereals with a little added salt.

- Sugar is simply carbohydrate that fuels your muscles. Yes, sugar calories are nutritionally empty calories. But when they are combined with lots of nutrients from the milk, banana, juice, and cereal itself, the twenty empty calories in five grams of added sugar are insignificant. Obviously, sugar-filled frosted flakes and kids' cereals with ten grams of sugar or more per serving are somewhat more like dessert than breakfast. Hence, try to limit your breakfast choices to cereals with fewer than five grams of added sugar per serving. Eat the sugary ones for snacks or dessert, if desired.

4. *Choose primarily low-fat cereals with less than two grams of fat per serving.*

High-fat cereals such as some brands of granola and crunchy cookie-type cereals can add unexpected fat and calories to your sports diet. Select low-fat brands for the foundation of your breakfast, then use only a sprinkling of the higher-fat treats, if desired, for a topping.

I'm not hungry in the morning: If you have no morning appetite, the chances are you ate your breakfast calories the night before. Huge dinner? Ice cream? Too many cookies before bedtime? The solution to having no morning appetite is, obviously, to eat less at night so that you can start the day off hungry.

If running first thing in the morning "kills your appetite" (due to the rise in body temperature), keep in mind that you *will* be hungry within a few hours when you have cooled down. Plan ahead, so when the hungry horrors hit, you will have healthful brunch options ready and waiting. Otherwise, you'll be likely to grab whatever's easy, which may include doughnuts, pastries, cookies, and other high-fat foods.

I'm on a diet: Too many weight-conscious people start their diet at breakfast. Bad idea. Breakfast skippers tend to gain weight and to be heavier than breakfast eaters. A satisfying breakfast *prevents you from getting too hungry* and overeating.

Your best bet for successful dieting is to *eat during the day*, burn off the calories, and then eat a light meal at night. Chapter 14 has more details about how to lose weight and have energy to train.

Breakfast makes me hungrier: Many marathoners complain that if they eat breakfast, they seem to get hungrier and eat more all day. This may result from thinking they have already "blown their diets" by eating breakfast, so they might as well keep overeating, then start dieting again the next day. Wrong.

Successful diets start at breakfast. If you feel hungry after breakfast you probably *ate too little* breakfast. For example, 100 calories of toast with jam is enough to whet your appetite but not to satisfy your calorie needs. Try budgeting about one-third of your calories for breakfast and/or a mid-morning snack—500–600 calories for most 120–150 pound runners. This translates into two slices of toast with jam, a banana, low-fat yogurt, *and* juice; or yogurt and a bagel with peanut butter.

Note: If you *over*eat at breakfast, you can easily resolve the problem by eating less at lunch or dinner. You won't be as physically hungry for those meals and will be able to easily eat smaller portions.

● **THE BREAKFAST OF CHAMPIONS**—By now, I hope I've convinced you that breakfast is indeed the most important meal of the day for marathoners. *What* should you eat, you wonder? If you feel like cooking, enjoy hot oatmeal, French toast, or pancakes.

But if you are looking for a cook-free choice, I highly recommend cereal. Cereal is quick, convenient, and filled with the calcium, iron, carbohydrates, fiber, and other nutrients active people need. A bowl of bran cereal with fruit and low-fat milk provides

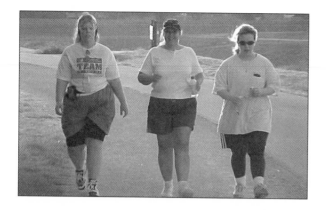

Breakfast is particularly important for people who walk or run
in the morning. Exercising on
an empty stomach may leave
you lagging in energy.

a well-balanced meal that includes three of the five food groups (grain, milk, and fruit) and sets the stage for an overall low-fat diet.

Cereal is versatile. You can eat it dry if you're on the run, or preferably with low-fat milk and/or yogurt for a calcium booster. You can mix brands and vary the flavor with different toppings:

- sliced banana
- blueberries (a handful of frozen ones taste great—especially if microwaved)
- raisins
- canned fruit
- cinnamon
- maple syrup
- vanilla yogurt

" I still find it hard to believe that when I started eating more at breakfast and lunch, I lost weight. I felt as though I was cheating all the time. My running times even improved because I was actually well-fueled instead of half-starved. "

Laura Perkins, New York City, NY

My personal favorite is to put a mix of cereals in my bowl, top it with fruit, heat it in the microwave oven for 30 to 60 seconds, and then add cold milk. It's like eating fruit cobbler!

● **SUMMARY**—What you eat in the morning provides fuel for more energy and stronger workouts. Breakfast helps novice and experienced marathoners alike to make their way to the winners' circle! Even dieters can enjoy breakfast without the fear of "getting fat"—that is, breakfast helps curb evening appetite so that dieters can eat lighter at night.

If you generally skip breakfast, at least give breakfast a try during your marathon training. You'll soon learn why breakfast is the meal of champions!

Oatmeal Pancakes

These pancakes are light and fluffy prizewinners, perfect for carbo-loading or recovering from a long run.

½ cup oatmeal, uncooked

½ cup plain yogurt or buttermilk

½ to ¾ cup milk

1 egg or substitute

1 tablespoon oil, preferably canola

2 tablespoon firmly packed brown sugar

¼ teaspoon salt, as desired

1 teaspoon baking powder

½ teaspoon baking soda

1 cup flour, preferably half white, half whole-wheat

Optional:

dash cinnamon

1 cup blueberries

¼ cup sunflower seeds

1. In a medium bowl, combine the first three ingredients. Set the bowl aside for 15 to 20 minutes. This allows the oatmeal to soften.

2. When the oatmeal is through soaking, beat in the egg and oil, and mix well. Add the sugar, salt, and cinnamon, then the baking powder, baking soda, and flour.

3. Heat a large nonstick or lightly oiled skillet over medium heat.

4. For each pancake, pour about ⅓ cup of batter onto the skillet. Cook pancakes until the edges are slightly dry, and bubbles and holes form on top, about 2 minutes, being careful not to overcook the bottom. Flip each cake and continue cooking until lightly browned.

Serve with maple syrup or other topping of your choice.

YIELD:	6 six-inch pancakes
Total calories:	1,000
Calories per serving: (2 pancakes)	300

	Grams	% of calories
CARB	52	65
PRO	13	15
FAT	8	20

With 2 tablespoons of maple syrup: add 120 calories and 12 grams of carbohydrates.

Banana Bread

Whenever I have bananas that are getting too ripe, I'll make a loaf of banana bread. It makes a quick but hearty breakfast, lunch, or snack. Add some peanut butter and a glass of low-fat milk for a well-balanced meal and energy for the long run.

3 large bananas, the riper the better

1 egg or 2 egg whites

2 tablespoons oil, preferably canola

⅓ to ½ cup sugar

¼ cup milk

1 teaspoon salt, as desired

1 teaspoon baking soda

½ teaspoon baking powder

1½ cups flour, preferably half white, half whole-wheat

Preheat oven to 350°.

1. In a large bowl, mash the bananas with a fork. Add the egg, oil, sugar, milk, and salt. Beat well, then add the baking soda and baking powder.

2. Gently blend the flour into the banana mixture. Stir for 20 seconds or until just moistened.

3. Spray a 9x5-inch loaf pan with cooking spray. Pour the batter into the prepared pan.

Bake at 350° for 45 minutes or until a toothpick inserted near the middle comes out clean.

YIELD:	1 loaf, 12 slices
Total calories:	1,600
Calories per slice:	140

	Grams	% of calories
CARB	24 gm	70
PRO	3 gm	10
FAT	3 gm	20

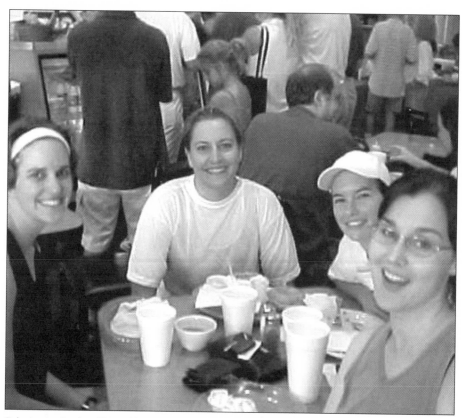

Enjoying a nice breakfast with training partners is one of the pleasures of marathoning. Be sure to include time for enjoyment of meals in your pre-marathon schedule.

CHAPTER 3

Lunch, Snack, and Dinner Ideas

L UNCH: THE SECOND MOST IMPORTANT MEAL OF THE DAY— Whereas breakfast is the most important meal of your training diet, lunch is the second most important. Brown-bagging it is a good way to save money, time, and sometimes calories if you are organized enough to pack your own lunch. Because of busy schedules, few marathoners make the effort to organize their lunch plans in advance of noontime (see sidebar: Brown-bag Lunches, page 23). Hence, fast foods can save the day... or do they spoil your sports diet?

• **FAST-FOOD LUNCHES**—The good news is that most quick-service restaurants now offer more low-fat foods than ever before. But, you'll likely be confronted by the many temptations that jump out at you while the healthier choices fade into the background. Before succumbing to grease, remind yourself that you will feel better and *feel better about yourself* if you eat well. Then, make the lower-fat choices:

Dunkin' Donuts: Low-fat muffins, bagels, juices, bean or broth-based soups, hot cocoa

Deli: Bagels; vegetable, bean or broth-based soups; sandwiches or subs with lots of bread and half the filling, little or no mayonnaise (Or ask for two extra slices of bread or a second roll to make a sandwich for tomorrow's lunch with the excessive meat.)

McDonald's: Grilled chicken sandwich with wholesome fluids such as juices, and low-fat milk

The following suggestions may help you pack a super sports lunch.

- To reduce chaos in your morning rush hour, make your lunch the night before.
- To prevent sandwich bread from getting stale, keep in it the freezer and take out the slices as needed. Bread thaws in minutes at room temperature, or in seconds in the microwave oven.
- Make several sandwiches at one time, then store them in the freezer. The frozen sandwich will be thawed—and fresh—by lunch time. Sliced turkey, lean roast beef, peanut butter, and leftover pizza freeze nicely. Don't freeze eggs, mayonnaise, jelly, lettuce, tomatoes, or raw veggies.
- Instead of eating a dry sandwich with no mayonnaise, add moistness using:
  - low-fat or fat-free mayonnaise
  - plain yogurt or yogurt/mayonnaise mixtures
  - low-fat or fat-free bottled salad dressings, such as ranch or creamy Italian
  - mustard and ketchup
  - salsa
  - lettuce and tomato
- Experiment:
  - peanut butter with sliced banana, raisins, dates, sunflower seeds, apple slices, and/or celery slices
  - cheese (preferably low-fat or a mixture of fat-free and regular) with oregano, Italian seasonings, green peppers, and/or tomatoes
- Pack leftover soups, chili, and pasta dinners for the next day's lunch. You can either eat the leftovers cold, or else heat them in the office microwave oven.

Wendy's:	Bowl of chili with a plain baked potato
Taco Bell:	Bean burrito
Pizza:	Thick-crust with extra veggies rather than extra cheese or pepperoni
Pasta:	Spaghetti or ziti with tomato sauce and a glass of low-fat milk for protein. Be cautious of lasagna, tortellini, or manicotti that are cheese-filled (i.e., high fat).
Chinese:	Hot and sour or wonton soup; plain rice with stir-fried entrées such as beef and broccoli or chicken with pea pods. Request the food be cooked with minimal oil. Limit fried appetizers and fried entrées.

Salads, whether served as a main dish or an accompaniment, are a simple way to boost your intake of fresh vegetables. The keys to making a healthy salad are:

- Use fresh vegetables.
- Choose a variety of colorful vegetables—dark green lettuces, red tomatoes, yellow peppers, orange carrots—for a variety of vitamins and minerals.
- Monitor the dressing. Some marathoners drown 50 calories of healthful salad ingredients with 400 calories of fatty dressing!

Here are how some popular salad ingredients compare. Note that the ones with the most color have the most nutritional value.

Salad Ingredient	Vitamin C (mg)	Vitamin A (IU)	Magnesium (mg)
Daily Value	60 mg	5,000 IU	400 mg
Broccoli, 5" stalk	110	2,500	24
Green pepper, ½	65	210	20
Spinach, 2 cups raw	50	8,100	90
Tomato, medium	35	1,400	20
Romaine, 2 cups	20	1,900	20
Iceburg, 2 cups	5	330	10
Cucumber, ½ medium	5	125	5
Celery, 1 stalk	5	120	10

Remember: You are better off having a substantial lunch than a huge dinner. Save the popular light, salad-type lunch for the evening meal.

● **THE FOUR O'CLOCK MUNCHIES**—In many countries such as England or Germany, the natives enjoy an afternoon cup of coffee or tea along with a sweet. This scheduled meal in their day provides a pleasant break as well as an energy booster. In comparison, many Americans believe eating in the afternoon is sinful. They self-inflict "Thou shalt not snack" as an Eleventh Commandment. Then, they succumb and feel guilty.

As I have mentioned before, hunger is not bad nor wrong. Hunger is simply your body's request for fuel. It is a normal physiological function. You can *expect* to get hungry every 4 hours. For example, if you eat lunch at noon, you can appropriately be hungry by 4:00. Eat something! If you are craving

The trick to making a substantial sports salad that's hearty enough to count as a meal is to add extra carbohydrates:

- dense vegetables, such as corn, peas, beets, carrots
- beans and legumes, such as chick-peas, kidney beans, and three-bean salad
- cooked rice or pasta
- oranges, apples, raisins, grapes
- toasted croutons
- whole-grain bread on the side

If you choose to use regular dressings, try to select ones made with olive oil for the flavor and the health-protective monounsaturated fats. If you want to reduce your fat intake, simply dilute regular dressings with water, more vinegar, or even milk (in ranch and other mayonnaise-based dressings). Or, choose from the plethora of low-fat and fat-free salad dressings available in stores and even salad bars. The commercial low-fat and fat-free dressings are good not only for salads, but also sandwiches, baked potatoes, and dips.

If you know the salad vegetables you buy will soon be wilting in your refrigerator, consider salad bars at the grocery store and deli as an easy and economical alternative to preparing your own.

sweets, you have gotten *too* hungry and should have eaten more food earlier.

Snacking is particularly important for dieters. As I will discuss in chapter 14, a *planned* afternoon snack of 100 to 400 calories (or whatever fits into your calorie budget) will prevent extreme hunger and reduce the risk of blowing your diet.

Outrageous snacks: If it's an ice cream sundae (or other such belt-busting treat) that you're craving, I recommend you satisfy your hankering by indulging at lunchtime. By spending your lunchtime calories on the treat, you can still balance your day's calorie budget and you'll certainly have incentive to run harder that afternoon. You also won't destroy your health with this occasional treat, as long as your overall diet tends to be wholesome.

Vending machine snacks: Vending-machine cuisine offers tough choices. Tucked between the lackluster choices, you may be able to find pretzels, peanuts, juice, yogurt, or even an apple. The good part about vending-machine snacks is that they are limited in size (e.g., only three cookies instead of the whole bag) and generally provide only 200 to 400 calories, not 2,000.

If trying to decide between fatty or sugary choices (i.e., chips v. jelly beans), remember that the sugar in jelly beans will appropriately fuel your muscles, whereas the fat in the chips will clog the arteries. After eating a sugary snack, be sure to brush or rinse your teeth.

● **DINNER AND MARATHONERS**—Dinnertime generally marks the end of the work day, a time to relax and enjoy a pleasant meal, that is, if you have the energy to prepare it. The trick to dining on a balanced dinner—the protein-starch-vegetable kind

---

● SOME SUPER SPORT SNACKS

The best sports snacks include *wholesome* carbohydrates. If you *carry snacks with you*, you can avoid the temptations that lurk in every corner store, vending machine, or bakery. Or keep a supply of "emergency food" in your desk drawer to be ready and waiting for the 4 o'clock munchies.

Nonperishable snacks to keep stocked:
- cold cereal (by the handful right out of the box or in a bowl with milk)
- hot cereal (packets of instant oatmeal are easy)
- pretzels
- reduced-fat microwave popcorn
- low-fat crackers
- peanut butter
- animal crackers
- low-fat granola bars
- energy bars
- noodle soups
- juice boxes
- dried fruit
- nuts
- trail mix

Perishable snacks:
- whole-wheat bagels
- English muffins
- Low-fat bran muffins
- microwaved potato
- low-fat yogurt
- thick-crust pizza
- fresh fruit
- leftover pasta

If you keep these foods stocked in your kitchen, you will have the makings for at least a week of simple meals:

- Spaghetti and tomato sauce, hamburger, ground turkey, tofu, beans, cottage cheese, grated cheese, and vegetables.
- English muffin or pita pizzas
- Tuna noodle casserole
- Soup and sandwiches (tuna, toasted cheese, peanut butter with banana)
- Microwaved potato topped with cottage cheese, baked beans, or yogurt
- Peanut butter crackers and V-8 juice
- Bean burritos

Cupboard: cereal, spaghetti, spaghetti sauce, (brown) rice, ramen noodles, (whole-grain) crackers, kidney beans, baked beans, refried beans, tuna, peanut butter, soups (mushroom for making casseroles, lentil, minestrone, hearty bean), baking potatoes, V-8 or other vegetable juices.

Refrigerator: low-fat Cheddar, mozzarella and cottage cheese, low-fat milk and yogurt, Parmesan cheese, eggs, tofu, tortillas, carrots, lettuce, tomatoes, oranges, bananas (when refrigerated, the banana peel turns black but the fruit itself is fine and lasts longer).

Freezer: whole-grain bagels, whole-wheat pita, English muffins, multigrain bread, orange juice concentrate, broccoli, spinach, winter squash, ground turkey, extra-lean hamburger, chicken (pieces frozen individually in baggies).

that mom used to make with at least three kinds of foods—is to arrive home with enough energy to cook. This means fueling your body and brain with adequate calories prior to the dinner hour. If you are cooking-challenged, you might want to take a cooking class at your local center for adult education. But no number of cooking classes will help if you arrive home too hungry to cook or make wise food choices.

● **QUICK FIXES: DINNER TIPS FOR HUNGRY RUNNERS**—Because good nutrition starts in the supermarket, you have a far better chance of achieving a super sports diet when your kitchen is well stocked with appropriate foods. You might want to muster up your energy to marathon shop at the discount or warehouse food store once every two or three weeks and really shop, so that you have enough food to last for a while. To help accomplish this goal, post a copy of the sidebar: *Runner's Basic Shopping List* (page 27) on your refrigerator and check off the foods you need.

If possible, you can use your morning shower/shave time to cook a potful of rice while getting ready for work. Come dinner time, you can simply brown hamburger or ground turkey in a large skillet, dump in the cooked rice, and then add whatever is handy. The ratio of 1½ cups raw rice per pound of raw lean meat results in two generous sports meals with 60 percent of the calories from carbohydrates. Some popular creations with rice and ground meat include:

- *Mexican* – canned beans + chili powder + grated low-fat Cheddar cheese + diced tomatoes
- *Chinese* – broccoli zapped in the microwave oven while the meat cooks + soy sauce
- *Italian* – green beans + Italian seasonings such as basil, oregano, and garlic powder
- *American* – grated low-fat Cheddar cheese + onion browned with the meat + diced tomatoes

Here are some ideas for quick and easy meals:
- pasta with clam sauce, tomato sauce, and/or frozen vegetables, and/or low-fat cheese
- canned beans, rinsed and then spooned over rice, pasta, or salads
- frozen dinners, supplemented with whole-grain bread and fresh fruit
- Pierogies, tortellini, and burritos from the frozen food section
- baked potato topped with cottage cheese
- whole-grain cereal (hot or cold) with fruit and low-fat milk
- thick-crust pizza, fresh or frozen, then reheated in the toaster oven
- bean soups, homemade, canned, or from the deli
- quick-cooking brown rice—made double for the next day's rice and bean salad
- stir-fry, using pre-cut vegetables from the market, salad bar, or freezer

> **I've never been as hungry as I was in the months before my marathon. I found the only way to stay pleasant was to make sure I always had a snack nearby—apples, energy bars, and baby carrots.**
>
> Amy Singer, Seattle, WA

One of the nicest things about making homemade soups and stews is having their aroma fill the house. What a wonderful greeting upon returning from a long winter run! I like to keep soups and stews on hand for quick evening meals that simply need to be heated. A bowl of warm soup is a relatively effortless dinner, thanks to the microwave oven.

If you frequently make soups or stews, you might want to:

- Save the cooking water from vegetables in a jar in the refrigerator to use as a soup base.
- Limit the seasonings so that you can add the seasoning-of-the-day into the individual portion you will be eating. That way, you can have Chinese-style soup one day, curried soups another, and Mexican a third.

There is nothing wrong with using canned soups or broths for the foundation of a quick and easy meal. Because the canned products tend to have more sodium than do some homemade soups and stews, runners with high blood pressure should choose the low-sodium canned soups.

Here are some ways to convert plain ol' canned soup into a more exotic meal, light supper, or snack:

- *Combine soups*
  - onion and chicken noodle
  - tomato and vegetable

- *Add ingredients*
  - diced celery, broccoli, tomatoes, or whatever fresh or frozen vegetable is handy
  - leftover rice, noodles, pasta
  - leftover vegetables, salads, casseroles
  - whatever in the 'fridge needs to be eaten

- *Add seasonings*
  - curry powder to chicken soup
  - cloves to tomato soup
  - wine, sherry, vermouth to mushroom soup

- *Add toppings*
  - Parmesan cheese
  - grated low-fat cheeses
  - cottage cheese
  - sesame seeds
  - croutons

● **PASTA: A SUPERFOOD?**—Every marathoner regardless of language understands the word *pasta*. Pasta parties are universally enjoyed around the world. Pasta is popular not only pre-marathon, but also as a standard part of the training diet. Even marathoners who claim they can't cook manage to boil pasta in one shape or another. Some choose to eat pasta at least five nights of the week thinking it is a kind of superfood.

Granted, pasta is carbohydrate-rich, quick and easy to cook,

If you have the choice between plain pasta or potato for dinner, consider the potato. It offers far more vitamin C, potassium, fiber, and overall health value. A potato is even better than rice, and a sweet potato the best of all. Here's the lineup for these popular dinner starches:

Food/Amount	Calories	Vitamin C (mg)	Potassium (mg)	Thiamin (mg)	Fiber (g)
Spaghetti, plain 2 cups cooked; ¼ lb. dry	420	0	85	0.5	4
Spaghetti, 100% whole wheat 2 cups cooked; ¼ lb. dry	420	0	150	0.4	16
Brown rice 2 cups cooked; ½ cup dry	420	0	165	0.4	7
Potato, plain baked, with skin 2 large; 15 oz. total wt.	420	52	1,700	0.4	10
Sweet potato, baked, with skin 2 large; 15 oz. total wt.	420	100	1,400	0.3	12

heart-healthy, economical, fun to eat, and enjoyed by just about every member of the family. But in terms of vitamins, minerals, and protein, plain pasta is a lackluster food. Here's some information to help you to place pasta in perspective.

Nutritional Value: Pasta is an excellent source of carbohydrates for muscle fuel and is the equivalent of "gas" for your engine. But plain pasta is a marginal source of vitamins and minerals, the "spark plugs" you need for top performance. Pasta is simply made from refined white flour—the same stuff you get in "wonder breads"—with a few vitamins added to replace those lost during processing.

Note that whole-wheat pastas have substantial fiber but offer little nutritional superiority, because wheat (and other grains in general) are better respected for their carbohydrate-value than their vitamins and minerals. Even spinach and tomato pastas are often overrated since they contain relatively little spinach or tomato in comparison to having a serving of that vegetable along with the meal.

Plain pasta becomes more of a nutritional powerhouse when you top it with:

- tomato sauce rich in vitamins A and C and potassium
- pesto-type sauces rich in vitamins A and C and potassium
- clam sauce rich in protein, zinc, and iron.

Pasta can be an artery-clogging nutritional nightmare if you eat it smothered with butter, cream, or greasy meat sauces.

Pasta and Protein: Pasta is popular not only for carbohydrates but also for being a vegetarian alternative to meat-based meals. However, many marathoners live on *too much* pasta and neglect their protein needs. For example, Joe, an aspiring marathoner, thought his high-carbohydrate, low-fat diet of pasta and tomato sauce seven nights per week was top notch. He came to me wondering why he felt chronically tired and was not improving despite hard training.

The answer was simple. His limited diet was deficient in not only protein but also iron and zinc. Once he started to supplement the pasta with a variety of proteins, he started to feel better, run better, and recover better. He added to his tomato sauce a variety of protein-rich choices:
- 2–3 ounces of extra-lean ground beef or turkey:
- ¼ cup of grated low-fat mozzarella cheese
- ½ cake tofu
- ⅔ cup canned, drained kidney beans
- 3 ounces tuna (one-half of a 6-ounce can)
- ½ cup of clams
- 1 cup of low-fat cottage cheese

Or, instead of adding protein to the sauce, he drank two glasses of low-fat milk with the meal.

● **SUMMARY**—If you are like many marathoners who know what they "should" eat but just don't do it, you need to remember the following keys to a successful sports diet:
1. Eat appropriately sized meals on a regular schedule so that you won't get too hungry. Notice how your diet deteriorates when you get too hungry; you'll eat more snacks, fewer meals.
2. Spend your calories on a variety of wholesome foods at each meal. Target three kinds of food per meal.
3. Pay attention to how much better you feel, run, and feel about yourself when you eat a well-balanced sports diet.

Not everyone is a pasta fan. German and Irish runners are among the many who thrive on potatoes. Potatoes are pre-wrapped, convenient, nutritious, and a great source of carbohydrates, potassium, and vitamin C. A large baking potato offers 65 percent the recommended intake (the Daily Value) for vitamin C and all the potassium you'd lose in three hours of sweaty exercise. A sweet potato offers the additional health benefits of beta-carotene.

Baked potatoes are a good sports food for not only meals but also snacks. Some marathoners carry them in a pocket, as they might a piece of fruit, and munch on them during and after workouts when they need an energy booster.

To help you include more potatoes in your sports diet, here are some tips:

- Potatoes come in different varieties, with some varieties best suited for baking (russets), others for boiling (red or white rounds). Ask the produce manager at your grocery store for guidance.
- Potatoes are best stored in a cool, humid (but not wet) place that is well ventilated, such as your cellar. Do not refrigerate potatoes because they will become sweet and off-colored.
- Rather than peel the skin (under which is stored most of the vitamin C), scrub the skin well, cook it, and eat it, skin and all. Even mashed potatoes can be made unpeeled!
- One pound of potatoes = three medium = two large. The large "restaurant size" potato generally has about 200 calories.
- To bake a potato in the oven, allow about 40 minutes at 400° for a medium potato, closer to an hour for a large potato. Because potatoes can be baked at any temperature, you can simply adjust the cooking time to whatever else is in the oven.
- You can tell if the potato is done if you can easily pierce it with a fork.
- To cook a potato in the microwave oven, prick the skin in several places with a fork, place it on some paper towels in the bottom of the microwave, and cook it for about 4 minutes if it is medium-sized, 6 to 10 minutes if large. Cooking time will vary according to the size of the potato, the power of your oven, and the number of potatoes being cooked. Turn the potato over halfway through cooking. Remove the potato from the oven, wrap it in a towel and allow it to finish cooking for about 3 to 5 minutes.

It's my opinion that *getting too hungry is the biggest problem* with most marathoners' diets. Hearty carbohydrate-based meals set the stage for a top-notch sports diet.

Quick and Easy Baked Potato Ideas

To spice-up your potato, try the following toppings:

- Plain yogurt
- Imitation butter granules (such as Molly McButter) and milk
- Mustard
- Mustard and Worcestershire sauce
- Vinegar and flavored vinegars
- Soy sauce
- Pesto
- Chopped chives and green onion
- Herbs, such as dill, parsley, chopped chives
- Steamed broccoli or other cooked vegetables
- Chopped jalapeno peppers
- Low-fat or fat-free salad dressing
- Fat-free sour cream, chopped onion, and grated low-fat cheddar cheese
- Cottage cheese and garlic powder
- Cottage cheese and salsa
- Soup broth
- Milk mashed into the potato
- Lentils or lentil soup
- Applesauce

● SOUP RECIPE

Simple Winter Squash Soup for One

When you are hankering for something nourishing and sweet, this squash soup will do the job with wholesome carbohydrates rich in beta-carotene. To make this soup into a more substantial meal, simply add some cooked ground turkey and/or leftover rice.

1 10-ounce package frozen winter squash

1 cup milk

2 to 3 teaspoons brown sugar

1 teaspoon salt, as desired

Optional:

- a few dashes ginger or nutmeg
- cooked ground turkey
- leftover rice

1. In a saucepan or a microwaveable dish, heat the squash with the milk.

2. Add the brown sugar, salt, seasonings, and other add-ins, as desired. Stir until blended.

3. Pour into a bowl or mug, and enjoy.

YIELD:	1 serving
Total calories:	220

	Grams	% of calories
CARB	40	75
PRO	11	20
FAT	2	5

CHAPTER 4

Vitamins and Supplements for Marathoners

ITAMINS ARE ESSENTIAL SUBSTANCES THAT YOUR BODY CAN'T make. They perform important jobs in your body, including helping to convert food into energy. Because vitamin supplements seem to be growing in popularity (surveys suggest that 75–90 percent of athletes take some type of supplement), you may wonder if you should jump on the supplement bandwagon and begin taking them.

> ❝ **Vitamin pills are great, but there's no substitute for the real thing.** ❞
>
> Jonathan Dietrich, Washington, DC

Although a supplement is certainly quick and easy health insurance, I highly recommend that you first make the effort to "eat" your vitamins. As a hungry marathoner who requires more calories than the average person, you can easily consume large doses of all nutrients and potentially benefit from this bonus. Chapter 1 has information about the best food sources of vitamins.

Because food consumption surveys suggest that many people fail to eat a well-balanced variety of wholesome foods, some runners and walkers may indeed suffer from marginal nutritional deficiencies, particularly those who:

• restrict calories
• eat a repetitive diet of bagels and pasta
• skimp on fruits, vegetables, and dairy foods
• over-indulge in fats and sweets

Even marathoners who believe they eat well sometimes miss the mark. For example, one woman who took pride in her high-carbohydrate, low-fat diet (primarily bagels, bananas, pasta, and pretzels) ate too many carbohydrates at the exclusion of other foods (such as meats and dairy). She had a diet deficient in calcium, iron, zinc, and protein.

As a result of American's unbalanced food choices, should the general public be encouraged to take a supplement to compensate for poor eating habits? Not necessarily. Despite the rising popularity of supplements, most health professionals recommend food, not pills, for optimal nutrition. The key is to learn how to eat healthfully despite a hectic eat-and-run lifestyle. Let's take a look at some of what is and what is not known about nutritional supplements, and hopefully you'll see why spending more money on broccoli and spinach rather than on pills is the wiser bet.

Vitamins were originally studied to determine the minimal amount of a nutrient required to prevent deficiency diseases such as beriberi and scurvy. The recommended dietary allowances (RDAs) were developed to guide people towards an appropriate intake. The RDA includes a large safety margin. For example, the RDA for vitamin C is 60 milligrams, which is six times the minimal amount needed to prevent the deficiency disease scurvy. The question remains unanswered: What is the optimal level of vitamins, not just to prevent *deficiency*, but to *enhance* health?

No amount of any supplement will compensate for a high-fat, hit-or-miss diet and stress-filled lifestyle. Taking supplements can also down-play the value of *whole* foods that offer protein, carbohydrates, and fiber—far more than just vitamins and minerals. But supplements are indeed appropriate for certain populations, including:

• runners on low-calorie reduction diets
• pregnant women
• women who *might* become pregnant
  (expectedly or unexpectedly)
• vegetarians
• those who are sick and are not eating well
• seniors

To date, no studies have documented a physiological need for mega-doses of vitamins, even for marathoners and other athletes. Rather, the research indicates most athletes can consume more than enough vitamins through their daily food intake.

● **FOOD OFFERS MORE THAN VITAMINS**—Whole foods such as fruits and vegetables offer hundreds, perhaps thousands, of substances called *phytochemicals* that protect our health. These include:

- *protease inhibitors* in soybeans that may slow tumor growth
- *isoflavones* in dried beans that may reduce the risk of breast or ovarian cancer
- *isothiocyanates* in broccoli that may help block carcinogens from damaging a cell's DNA

These phytochemicals may explain why the cruciferous vegetables such as broccoli, cabbage, and cauliflower are thought to be protective against cancer, and onions and garlic are thought to be protective against heart disease.

As you decide your nutritional fate, know that a diet based on a variety of wholesome foods is your best source of good nutrition. If you choose to take a supplement for its potential health-protective effects, be sure to do so *in addition to eating well*. The anti-oxidant vitamins (C, beta-carotene, and E) show the most promise. Although you can get sufficiently large amounts of C and beta-carotene (and phytochemicals) from fruits and vegetables, you likely need a supplement to get an effective dose of E (100 to 400 IU). Because researchers have yet to unravel the whole vitamin/health mystery, stay tuned and be sure to take care of your whole health. The phytochemicals and perhaps other unknown substances found in whole foods, but not in pills, may emerge as the winner.

● **AM I SICK? AM I TIRED? DO I NEED VITAMINS?**—Exercise energizes many people, enhancing their productivity as well as relieving their stress. But some marathoners complain of chronic fatigue. They feel run down, dragged out, and overwhelmingly exhausted. If this sounds familiar, you may wonder if you are sick, overtired, or if something is wrong with your diet. You may wonder if taking vitamins would solve the problem.

Perhaps you can relate to Peter, a 39-year-old marathon runner, lawyer, and solo-chef who bemoaned, "I just don't take the time to eat right. My diet is awful. I rarely eat fruits or vegetables, to say nothing of a real meal. I think that poor nutrition is catching up with me. What vitamins should I take?"

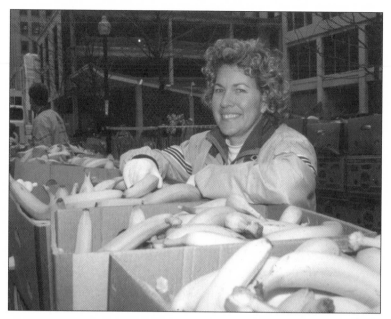

No amount of vitamin pills can compensate for a lack of fruits and vegetables. Eat up!

Peter lived alone, hated to cook for just himself, tended to survive on fast (and fatty) foods. He rarely ate breakfast, barely ate lunch, but always collapsed after a long day with a generous feast of a large deli sandwich, Chinese take-out, or pizza. He struggled to wake up in the morning, to stay awake during afternoon meetings, and to grind through his daily ten-mile run.

I evaluated Peter's diet, calculated that he had 3,000 calories in his daily energy budget (1,000 calories per section of the day—that is, morning, afternoon, and evening), and suggested a few simple food changes that could result in higher energy, greater stamina, and better running. Trying to find some solutions to Peter's fatigue, I explored the following questions. Perhaps the answers will offer solutions for your energy problems.

- *Are you tired due to low blood sugar?* Peter skipped not only breakfast but also often missed lunch because he "didn't have time." He would doze off in the afternoon because he had low blood sugar. With zero calories to feed his brain, he ended up feeling sleepy.

  The solution was to *choose* to make time to eat. Just as he chose to sleep later in the morning, he could choose to get up five minutes earlier for breakfast; he could also choose to stop working for five or ten minutes to eat lunch.

- *Is your diet too low in carbohydrates?* Peter's fatty food choices filled his stomach but left his muscles poorly fueled with inadequate glycogen to support his training program. Higher carb snacks and meals would not only fuel his muscles but also help maintain a higher blood sugar level thereby providing energy for mental work as well as physical exercise.

- *Are you iron-deficient and anemic?* Peter ate little red meat and consequently little iron, an important mineral in red blood cells that helps carry oxygen to exercising muscles. Iron-deficiency anemia can result in needless fatigue during exercise. I taught Peter how to boost his dietary iron intake, with or without meat. (See Chapter 5.) I also recommended blood tests (hemoglobin, hematocrit, ferritin, serum iron, and total iron-binding capacity) to rule out the question of anemia.

- *Are you getting enough sleep?* Peter's complaint about being chronically tired was justified because he was tired both mentally (from his intense job) and physically (from his strenuous training). He worked from 8 A.M. to 8 P.M. By the time he got home, ran, ate dinner, and "unwound," midnight had rolled around. The wake-up bell at 6:30 A.M. came all too soon—especially since Peter often had trouble falling asleep due to having eaten such a large dinner.

  I recommended that Peter try to get more sleep by eating lighter dinners (soup and sandwich, or even cereal), having bigger breakfasts, and scheduling his main meal at lunch (low-fat Chinese meals, pizza, or pasta). By trading in 1,200 of his evening calories for 600 more calories at breakfast and 600 more calories at lunch, he could determine if less food in his stomach before bed would result in better sleep.

- *Are you overtraining?* Although Peter took pride in the fact that he hadn't missed a day of running in seven years, he felt discouraged he wasn't improving despite harder training. I questioned whether he was a "compulsive runner" who punished his body or a "serious athlete" who trained wisely and took rest days. One or two rest days or easy days per week are an essential part of a training program; they allow the body to replenish its depleted muscle glycogen.

- **Are you stressed or depressed?** Peter not only had a stressful job, he was also dealing with the stress and depression associated with family problems, to say nothing of the challenges of training for a marathon. Since he was feeling a bit helpless with this situation, I encouraged him to successfully control at least one aspect of his life—his diet. Simple dietary improvements could not only help him feel physically better but also mentally better about himself. This would be very energizing in itself.

If you answered "yes" to many of the questions I asked Peter, you may be able to resolve your fatigue with better eating, sleeping, and training habits—not with vitamin pills. Experiment with the simple food suggestions in this book. Before long you may transform your current low-energy patterns into a food plan for success! Eating well is not as hard as you may think.

- **SUMMARY**—Your best bet for fighting fatigue is to nourish your body with the right balance of wholesome foods. Make the effort to eat a variety of foods and fluids from the different food groups every day. Eating marathoner's portions, you will consume not only the amounts of the vitamins and minerals you need, you will also be giving your body the *calories* it needs to prevent fatigue.

If you are tempted to take supplements as a type of health insurance, do so only if you simultaneously choose to eat a healthful diet. Remember, no amount of supplements will compensate for an inadequate diet—but you will *always* win with good nutrition. Eat wisely, eat well!

● SUPPLEMENT SAVVY

Confusion abounds regarding dietary supplements, their safety, and their potential health benefits. The FDA's Center for Food Safety and Applied Nutrition has a website to help answer your questions. Go to www.cfsan.fda.gov and click on *Dietary Supplements*.

CHAPTER 5

Protein for Marathoners

HISTORICALLY, PROTEIN WAS THE FUNDAMENTAL PART OF A SPORTS diet, thought to give power and strength. That's why some marathoners used to eat steak and eggs for their pre-marathon breakfast! Today we know these types of animal proteins do a poor job of fueling muscles but a good job of increasing the intake of saturated fats and the risk of heart disease.

Although too much protein offers no benefits to a sports diet, adequate protein is essential. About 10 to 15 percent of your calories should come from protein to:
• build and repair muscles
• make red blood cells
• make enzymes and hormones
• grow hair and fingernails.

Most marathoners, being health conscious, have heard the public health messages to eat less meat and have appropriately reduced their intake of it. But some marathoners have taken that advice to the extreme. They have totally cut out meats but have failed to add any plant proteins. The result is a protein-deficient diet.

If you aspire to a vegetarian diet and have stopped eating meat, make sure you are addressing your overall protein needs. Also recognize that being a vegetarian may require lifestyle changes. Pay attention to the flip side of your higher-carbohydrate diet by eating a small amount of protein-containing food at each meal. Otherwise, you'll feel the results of your dietary imbalance: chronic fatigue, anemia, lack of improvement,

Here a few ideas to help you with a meat-free diet that has adequate protein.

Breakfast:
- Cold cereal (preferably iron-enriched, as noted on the label): Add milk, yogurt, or soymilk, and sprinkle with a few nuts.
- Oatmeal, oat bran, and other hot cereals: Add peanut butter, almonds or other nuts, and/or powdered milk.
- Toast, bagels: Top with low-fat cheese, cottage cheese, or peanut butter.

Snacks:
- Assorted nuts
- Peanut butter on rice cakes or crackers
- Yogurt (Note: Frozen yogurt has only 4 grams of protein per cup, as compared to 8 grams of protein per cup of regular yogurt.)

Lunch and Dinner:
- Salads: Add tofu, chick peas, three-bean salad, marinated kidney beans, cottage cheese, sunflower seeds, chopped nuts.
- Protein-rich salad dressing: Add salad seasonings to plain yogurt, or blenderized tofu or cottage cheese (diluted with milk or yogurt).
- Spaghetti sauce: Add diced tofu and/or canned, drained kidney beans.
- Pasta: Choose protein-enriched pastas that offer 13 grams of protein per cup, as compared to 8 grams in regular pasta. Top with grated part-skim mozzarella cheese.
- Potato: Bake or microwave, then top with canned beans, baked beans, or low-fat cottage cheese.
- Hearty soups: Choose lentil, split pea, bean, and minestrone.
- Hummus: Try hummus with pita or tortillas.
- Cheese pizza: A protein-rich fast food, half of a 12-inch pizza has about 40 grams of protein.

muscle wasting, and an overall run-down feeling. Note that a protein-deficient diet can also lack iron (prevents anemia) and zinc (helps with healing). These minerals will be discussed later.

● **HOW MUCH PROTEIN IS ENOUGH?**—The current recommended dietary allowance (RDA) for protein is 0.4 grams of protein per pound of body weight (0.8 gm/kg). This RDA was based on *sedentary* college students. Because marathoners have a slightly higher

If you wonder if you are eating too little (or too much) protein, you can estimate your daily protein needs by multiplying your weight by 0.5 to 0.75 grams of protein per pound.

Weight	Protein
(pounds)	(grams per day)
100	50–80
120	60–90
150	75–100
170	85–115

Use food labels and the following chart to calculate your protein intake. Pay close attention to portion sizes!

Protein Content of Some Commonly Eaten Foods

Animal Proteins	Protein (grams)
Beef, 4 ounces cooked*	25
Chicken breast, small cooked	30
Tuna, 1 can (6.5 ounces)	40
Meat, fish, poultry, 1 ounce cooked	7
Egg, 1	7
Egg white, 1	3

Plant Proteins	
Lentils, beans, ½ cup	7
Baked beans, ½ cup	8
Peanut butter, 2 tablespoons	8
Tofu, ¼ cake (4 ounces)	7
Soy milk, 1 cup	7

Dairy Products	Protein (grams)
Milk, yogurt, 1 cup	8
Cheese, 1 ounce	8
Cheese, 1 slice American ⅔ ounce	6
Cottage cheese, ⅓ cup	8
Milk powder, ¼ cup	8

Breads, Cereals, Grains	
Bread, 1 slice	2
Cold cereal, 1 ounce	2
Oatmeal, ⅓ cup dry, or ⅔ cup cooked	5
Rice, ⅓ cup dry, or 1 cup cooked	4
Pasta, 2 ounces dry, or 1 cup cooked	8

Starchy Vegetables	
Peas, carrots, ½ cup cooked	2
Corn, ½ cup cooked	2
Beets, ½ cup cooked	2
Winter squash, ½ cup	2
Potato, 1 small	2

Fruits, Watery Vegetables
Negligible amounts of protein.

Most fruits and vegetables have only small amounts of protein. They may contribute a total of 5 to 10 grams protein per day, depending on how much you eat.

*4 ounces cooked = size of deck of cards
4 ounces cooked = 5 to 6 ounces raw

protein need, an adequate and safe protein intake is 0.5 to 0.75 grams of protein per pound of body weight (1.0 to 1.5 gm/kg).

Growing teenagers, athletes building new muscles, marathoners doing lots of long runs, or dieters who restrict calories (which results in protein being used for fueling rather than maintaining muscles), should target the higher end of the protein range.

● **COMBINING BEANS AND GRAINS**—The key to eating a high quality vegetarian diet is to eat a variety of foods that contain a variety of the eight essential amino acids needed for building protein. Historically, vegetarians were instructed to combine the amino acids from beans, grains, legumes, and/or seeds *in the same meal* in order to enhance the quality of their diet. Today we know this time frame can be expanded. You can simply eat a variety of these foods over the course of the day. Some effective protein-rich foods to combine through-out the day include:

- *Grains + milk products:*
  bran muffin + yogurt
  cereal + milk
  pasta + cheese
- *Grains + beans and legumes (such as peanuts, lentils, kidney, pinto, lima and navy beans):*
  bran muffin + peanut butter
  pasta + tomato sauce with
     canned kidney beans
  brown bread + baked beans
- *Legumes + seeds:*
  hummus (chickpeas + sesame butter)
  tofu + sunflower seeds (stir-fried with
     vegetables)
- *Milk products + any food:*
  milk, yogurt, or cheese added to any meal
     or snack

● **RED MEAT: EAT OR AVOID...?**—Red meats such as beef and lamb are indisputably excellent

> ❝ *Be sure to include enough protein in your training diet! I used to eat too many carbs and too little protein, and my performance suffered. Now I make sure to include some chicken or fish with my salads for dinner, and dairy with my breakfast each day. Once I started to pay attention to my protein intake, my recovery after long runs improved dramatically.* ❞
>
> Kip Parker, Boston, MA

- Beans are not only a good source of protein, but also carbohydrates, B-vitamins (such as folic acid), and fiber. When added to an overall low-fat diet, they may help lower elevated blood cholesterol levels.

- If beans cause you intestinal problems, eat small amounts. If you cook your own beans, be sure to soak them long enough before cooking. You can also try Beano, a product that when added to beans helps reduce gas formation.

Bean ideas:
- Sauté garlic and onions in a little oil; add canned, drained beans (whole or mashed); heat together.

- Add beans to salads, spaghetti sauce, soups, and stews for a protein booster.

- In a blender, mix black beans, salsa and cheese. Heat in the microwave and use as a dip or on top of tortillas or potatoes.

(See Bean Dip recipe, page 50)

sources of high-quality protein. They are also rich in iron and zinc, two minerals important for optimal health and athletic performance. Some meat-eating marathoners sound a bit unsure or even apologetic when asked if they eat red meat. Somehow eating beef can seem out of vogue, and confusion abounds regarding the pros and cons of eating it.

If you wonder whether or not you should eat or avoid red meat, know that the answer is not a simple yes or no but rather a weighing of nutrition facts, ethical concerns, personal values, and dedication to making appropriate food choices. Yes, you can get the nutrients needed to support your sports program from non red-meat sources, but will you make the effort to do so? The following facts can help you decide if tucking two to four small (3–4 ounce) portions of red meat per week into your meals might enhance the quality of your diet.

Meat for protein: Animal foods are excellent sources of high-quality protein. But so are plant proteins—if you eat *enough* of them. Marathoners with big appetites can accomplish this more easily than calorie-conscious dieters. If you eat only a little peanut butter on a lunchtime sandwich and a sprinkling of garbanzo beans on a dinner salad, you likely fall short of meeting the approximate 50–70 grams of protein needed by active women and 70–90 grams of protein needed by men. (See sidebar: *How to Balance your Protein Intake*, page 42.)

Meat and cholesterol: Meat, like chicken, fish, and other animal products, contains cholesterol because cholesterol is a part of animal cells; plant cells contain no cholesterol. Most animal proteins have similar cholesterol values: 70–80 milligrams of cholesterol per four ounce serving of red meat, poultry, and fish.

Given that the American Heart Association recommends that healthy people with normal blood cholesterol levels eat less than 300 milligrams of cholesterol per day, small portions of red meat can certainly fit those requirements. People who know their blood cholesterol number can best make personalized dietary decisions about how much dietary cholesterol is appropriate for their bodies.

> **It is easy to get enough carbs, but getting enough protein makes a big difference in my day-to-day performance.**
>
> Jonathan Dietrich, Washington, DC

Note that the cholesterol content of meat is of less concern than the fat content. *Fatty* meats such as greasy hamburgers, pepperoni, juicy steaks, and sausage are the real dietary no-nos. Lean meats— London broil, extra-lean hamburger, top round roast beef—can fit into a heart-healthy sports diet in appropriate amounts.

Meat and iron: Adequate iron in your sports diet is important to prevent anemia. Without question, the iron in red meat is

---

● CHICKEN AGAIN?

If you are tired of yet another boring chicken breast, spice it up with one of these ideas:

- Spread with mustard and sprinkle with Parmesan cheese
- Spread with honey and sprinkle with curry powder
- Marinate for an hour or overnight in Italian dressing
- Spread with honey mustard

Place in baking pan (lined with foil for easy clean up) and bake uncovered at 350° for 20 to 30 minutes.

- The recommended intake for iron is 8 milligrams for men and 18 milligrams for women per day. Women have higher iron needs to replace the iron lost from menstrual bleeding. Women who are post-menopausal require only 8 milligrams of iron per day.
- Iron from animal products is absorbed better than that from plant products.
- A source of vitamin C at each meal enhances iron absorption.

Animal Sources (best absorbed)	Iron (mg)	Beans	Iron (mg)
		Kidney, ½ cup	2½
Beef, 4 ounces cooked	2	Tofu, ¼ cake	2
Pork, 4 ounces	1	**Grains**	
Chicken breast, 4 ounces	1	Cereal, 100% iron fortified	18
Chicken leg, 4 ounces	1½	Spaghetti, 1 cup cooked	2
Salmon, 4 ounces	1	Bread, 1 slice, enriched	1
Fruits		**Other**	
Prunes, 5	1	Molasses, blackstrap, 1 tablespoon	3½
Raisins, ⅓ cup	1	Wheat germ, ¼ cup	2
Vegetables			
Spinach, ½ cup cooked	3		
Broccoli, ½ cup cooked	1		

more easily absorbed than that in popular vegetarian sources of iron (e.g., beans, raisins, spinach). In a study of eighteen women runners who consumed the recommended dietary allowance for iron, eight of the nine women who ate no red meat (but did eat chicken and fish) had depleted iron stores as compared to only two of the nine red-meat eaters.

If you eat an iron-poor diet and are tempted to simply take an iron supplement, note that animal iron is absorbed better than the iron in a pill. But any iron is better than no iron.

Meat and zinc: Zinc is important for healing both the minor damage that occurs with daily training as well as major injuries and ailments. It is best found in iron-rich foods (e.g., red meat). Diets deficient in iron may then also be deficient in zinc. Like iron, the zinc in animal products is absorbed better than that in vegetable foods or supplements.

Meat and amenorrhea: Female runners who have amenorrhea and have stopped getting their menstrual period commonly eat no red meat. In one study, *none* of the amenorrheic runners ate red meat as compared to 44 percent of the runners with regular menses.

The question remains unanswered: Are these amenorrheic athletes simply protein deficient or is there a meat factor that affects the hormones involved with menstruation? Given that amenorrhea is a sign of poor health, athletes who do not menstruate should carefully evaluate the adequacy of their diets and acknowledge that red meat may reduce the higher risk of stress fractures that coincides with the loss of menses. Refer to chapter 16 for more information.

Hormones in meats: Fears abound regarding hormones given to cattle to enhance their growth. The U.S. Department of Agriculture claims the amount of hormones used is far less than one might get in the birth control pill, or even in a cup of coleslaw, for that matter. You can always buy "all-natural" meat to be on the safe side.

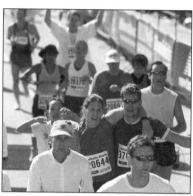

To get to the finish line, you need adequate protein as well as abundant carbohydrates.

● HOW TO BOOST YOUR ZINC INTAKE

- The recommended intake for zinc is 8 milligrams for women and 11 milligrams for men per day.
- Animal foods, including seafood, are the best sources of zinc.

Animal Sources	Zinc (mg)	Plant Sources	Zinc (mg)
Beef, tenderloin, 4 ounces	7	Wheat germ, ¼ cup	3.5
Chicken leg, 4 ounces	3.5	Lentils, 1 cup	2.5
Pork loin, 4 ounces	3	Almonds, 1 ounce	1
Chicken breast, 4 ounces	1	Garbanzo beans, ½ cup	1
Cheese, 1 ounce	1	Spinach, 1 cup cooked	0.7
Milk, 1 cup	1	Peanut butter, 1 tablespoon	0.5
Oysters, 6 medium	(!) 75	Bread, 1 slice, whole wheat	0.5
Tuna, 1 can (6½ ounces)	2		
Clams, 9 small	1		

Fish that are low in fat are also low in calories. But the fish that are high in fat offer better protection against heart disease. Here's the tally:

Fish (4 ounces cooked, or 6 ounces raw)	Calories	Protein (gm)	Fat (gm)
Bluefish	210	34	7
Catfish	200	31	7
Clams (8 large or 18 small)	130	22	2
Cod	140	30	1
Grouper	160	33	2
Haddock	150	32	1
Salmon, Atlantic	240	34	11
Salmon, sockeye	190	36	15
Shrimp (24 large)	180	35	3
Snapper	170	35	2
Swordfish	210	36	7
Tuna, fresh	240	40	8

Cooking with seafood is simple and a pleasure because of its versatility. You can bake, poach, steam, broil, stir-fry, and grill fish, depending on the type of fish. Nevertheless, many people shy away from seafood. My advice is to learn how to prepare fish because it is not only a great source of protein, but also of health-protective fish oils.

Here are some fish tips:
- Buy fresh fish that has no "fishy" odor. Ask to smell the fish before purchasing it. Fishy odor comes only with age and bacterial contamination.
- To rid your hands of any fishy smell, rub them with lemon juice or vinegar, then wash them.
- Seasonings that go well with fish include lemon, dill, basil, rosemary, and parsley (and paprika for color).
- Use the 10-minute rule for cooking fish: Cook fish 10 minutes per inch of thickness. Fold thin parts under to make the fish as even a thickness as possible. As fish cooks, the flesh turns from translucent to opaque white, similar to egg whites.
- To test for doneness, gently pull the fish apart with a fork. It should flake easily and no longer be translucent. Do not overcook fish. Perfectly cooked fish is moist and has a delicate flavor; overcooked fish is dry and tasteless.
- If possible, cook fish in its serving dish; fish is fragile and more attractive the less it is handled.

There are primarily two kinds of muscle fiber: *Fast-twitch* fibers are used for quick bursts of energy and *slow-twitch* fibers function best for endurance exercise. Elite marathon runners tend to have the right combination of both— a high proportion of slow-twitch fibers for the long run, but also enough fast-twitch fibers for the sprint to the finish.

The white and dark meat of chicken and turkey illustrate the difference between the two kinds of muscle: The white meat of the breast is primarily fast twitch; the dark meat of the legs, thighs, and wings is mostly slow twitch.

Slow-twitch muscles, more so than fast-twitch, rely on fat for fuel. This is why dark meat contains more fat than the white meat. On the plus side, dark meat also contains more nutrients—iron, zinc, and B-vitamins, many of the same nutrients found in red meats.

Chicken, without skin, 4 ounces cooked	Calories	Fat (gm)	Iron (gm)
Breast, white meat	180	4	1.2
Leg, dark meat	200	9	1.3
Thigh, dark meat	235	12	1.5

If you do not eat red meats, you might want to include more dark meat from chicken or turkey in your sports diet. For the small price of a few grams of fat, you'll get more nutritional value. If you want to cut back on fat, eliminate the skin—the fattiest part of poultry.

● **SUMMARY**—Marathoners who carefully select a vegetarian diet can certainly eat a high quality sports diet that meets their nutritional needs. However, marathoners who simply abstain from eating meat and make no effort to include alternate sources of protein, iron, and zinc should rethink their diet and reorganize their food choices. Or they might want to reconsider including small portions of lean meat two to four times per week as a convenient, nutrient-dense sports food. Remember that the *fat* in greasy meats, not the red meat itself, is the primary health culprit.

Bean Dip

This is good not only as a dip for (fat-free) tortilla chips, but also as a filling for tortillas. Add diced tomatoes and lettuce, if desired, to your tortilla before rolling it up.

1 16-ounce can vegetarian refried beans

1 16-ounce can vegetarian chili

6 ounces (1½ cups) grated low-fat Cheddar cheese

1. Spread the refried beans in the bottom of a shallow casserole dish or pie plate.
2. Add the vegetarian chili.
3. Sprinkle the cheese on top.
4. Heat in the microwave until bubbling.

YIELD:	10 servings
Total calories:	1,300
Calories per serving:	30

	Grams	% of calories
CARB	18	55
PRO	10	30
FAT	1	15

Creamy Fish Bake

1½ pounds halibut fillets or steaks (or other type of fish, as desired)

½ cup plain low-fat or fat-free yogurt

1 tablespoon reduced-fat or fat-free mayonnaise

2 tablespoons minced onion

1 teaspoons dried basil

Preheat oven to 400°.

1. Place the halibut in a baking pan.
2. In a small bowl, combine the remaining ingredients.
3. Spread the yogurt mixture over the halibut.
4. Bake uncovered at 400° for 10 to 15 minutes (depending on the thickness of the fish), until the fish flakes easily.

YIELD:	3 servings
Total calories:	960
Calories per serving:	320

	Grams	% of calories
CARB	5	5
PRO	57	70
FAT	8	25

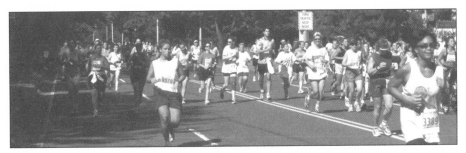

All runners, whether vegetarian or meat-eating, need adequate protein to build and protect their muscles as well as to recover from exhaustive exercise.

CHAPTER 6

Fats and Your Sports Diet

MANY MARATHONERS RESTRICT THEIR FAT INTAKE BECAUSE OF their desire to be healthy. This is a wise health practice that is often taken to the extreme. In this anti-fat era, some athletes think all they need to know about fat is that they are supposed to avoid it like the plague. Rumors abound:

• Fat instantly clogs the arteries or causes cancer.
• Fat slows you down; it's the worst food you could put in your body.
• If you eat fat, you'll get fat.

While there may be an element of truth in some of these statements, there is also room for more education. Let's look at the whole picture.

First of all, remember fat is an essential nutrient needed for overall good health. Whereas a little bit of fat is an appropriate part of your sports diet, too much fat leaves your muscles un-fueled. Without question, a diet saturated with animal fats, fast-food grease, and obscene desserts may also contribute to heart disease and cancer and shorten your life span. But if you are lean, fit, and healthy and have:

• low blood cholesterol (or high levels of the good HDL cholesterol)
• a family history of longevity
• no family history of heart disease

you can appropriately include a reasonable amount of fat in your diet. The people who most likely need to restrict their fat intake to less than 20 percent of calories are overfat, under-fit folks with heart disease—not most healthy walkers and runners.

I recommend that healthy marathoners target a sports diet with about 25 percent of the calories from fat. This:

- is in keeping with the 20 to 30 percent fat diet that is considered to be health-protective.
- allows for adequate carbohydrates (55–65 percent of total calories) and proteins (10–15 percent of total calories).
- provides fat-soluble vitamins such as vitamin E (an antioxidant that has a health-protective effect).
- allows for easier participation in life (i.e., eating at a party, enjoying a cookie guilt-free).

How does 25 percent fat translate into food? Let's say you have 1,800 calories a day in your calorie budget:

.25 x 1,800 total calories = 450 calories a day of fat.

Because there are 9 calories per gram of fat, divide 450 calories by 9:

450 calories/9 calories per gram = 50 grams of fat in your daily fat budget.

A 25-percent-fat diet includes a reasonable amount of fat and lets you enjoy a little fat at each meal. Preferably, you'll choose fats that have positive health value such as olive oil, canola oil, salmon and other oily fish, all-natural peanut butter, low-fat cheese, nuts, and tuna with light mayonnaise. But, if you do have the occasional hankering for a big burger with 25 grams of fat and 500 calories, simply fit it into your day's fat and calorie budget *and balance the rest of the day's meals.* (Refer to Chapter 13 to determine your calorie needs.)

● **FEAR OF FAT**—Without question, fat imparts a tempting taste, texture, and aroma and helps make food taste great. That's why fatty foods can be hard to resist and are enjoyed to *excess.* Although excess fat-calories can easily turn into body fat, note the "eat fat, get fat" theory is false. Many active people eat appropriate amounts of fat and stay thin. They simply don't *overeat* calories.

If you are weight-conscious and obsess about every gram

of fat to the extent you have a fat phobia, your fear of fat may be exaggerated! A little fat can actually aid in weight reduction because it adds *satiety*—the nice feeling of being satisfied after a meal. Satiety may actually *reduce* your desire to continue munching even after you've eaten your bulky but unfilling fat-free meal.

Believe it or not, many of my clients have lost body fat after they reintroduced an appropriate amount of dietary fat back into their fat-free regimen. Refer to the weight reduction information in Chapter 14 for additional help with resolving your "eat fat, get fat" fears.

Although all fats are equally caloric, some fats provide more health benefits than others. Olive oil, for one, is thought to be health-protective. It is the founda-tion of the acclaimed heart-healthy Mediterranean Diet.

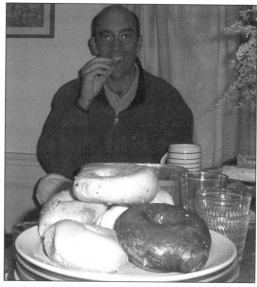

Spreading peanut butter on a bagel adds more protein and healthful fat than you'd get from cream cheese.

For centuries, the folks in Italy and Greece have enjoyed good health and a 40 percent fat diet. Their diet is rich in mono-unsaturated fat from olive oil, not saturated fat from greasy meats and lard. Olive oil in combination with the Mediterranean diet's bounty of beans, fresh seafood, fruits, and vegetables are all positive factors that may combine with phys-ically active lifestyles to enhance longevity.

● **SUMMARY**—Marathoners who include some fat in their daily training diet perform better than those who try to exclude fat. Obviously, choosing the *healthful* fats—olive oil, canola oil, nuts, peanut butter—is preferable to loading up on the fat from buttery cookies, greasy burgers, and gourmet ice cream. But *all* fats eaten in moderation can be balanced into an overall healthful and carbohydrate-rich sports diet.

FAT GUIDELINES

The following guidelines can help you appropriately budget fat into your food plan.

Calories per day	Fat grams per day (for 25-percent-fat diet)
1,600	45
1,800	50
2,000	55
2,200	60
2,400	65

Fat Content of Some Common Foods

Food	Serving size	Fat (grams)	Calories
Dairy products			
Milk, whole (3½% fat)	1 cup	8	150
Milk, reduced-fat (2% fat)	1 cup	5	120
Milk, low-fat (1% fat)	1 cup	2	100
Milk, fat-free (0% fat)	1 cup	—	80
Cheese			
Cheddar	1 ounce	9	110
Reduced-fat	1 ounce	5	90
Mozzarella, part-skim	1 ounce	5	80
Cottage cheese (4% fat)	½ cup	5	120
Low-fat cottage cheese (2% fat)	½ cup	2	90
Cream cheese	1 oz. (2 tbsp.)	10	100
Cream cheese, light	1 oz. (2 tbsp.)	5	60
Ice cream, gourmet	½ cup	15	250
Ice cream, standard	½ cup	8	150
Ice cream, light	½ cup	3	110
Frozen yogurt, low-fat	½ cup	2	120
Frozen yogurt, fat-free	½ cup	—	100
Animal proteins			
Beef, regular hamburger	4 oz. cooked	24	330
Beef, flank steak	4 oz. cooked	12	235
Beef, eye of round	4 oz. cooked	6	200
Chicken, breast, no skin	4 oz. cooked	5	200
Chicken, thigh, no skin	4 oz. cooked	11	235
Fish, haddock	4 oz. cooked	1	125
Fish, swordfish	4 oz. cooked	6	175

Food	Serving size	Fat (grams)	Calories
Vegetable proteins			
Beans, kidney	½ cup cooked	—	110
Lentils	½ cup cooked	—	110
Tofu	4 oz.	5	90
Peanut butter	1 tablespoon	8	95
Fats			
Butter	1 tablespoon	12	110
Margarine	1 tablespoon	11	100
Oil, olive	1 tablespoon	13	120
Mayonnaise	1 tablespoon	11	100
Grains			
Bread, whole wheat	1 large slice	1	90
Crackers, Saltines	5	2	60
Crackers, Ritz	4	4	70
Rice cakes	1	—	35
Cereal, shredded wheat	1 oz. (⅔ cup)	—	90
Cereal, granola	1 oz. (¼ cup)	6	130
Cereal, oatmeal	1 oz. (⅓ cup) dry	2	100
Spaghetti, plain	2 oz. dry (1 cup cooked)	1	210
Rice	2 oz. dry (1 cup cooked)	—	200
Fast foods			
Big Mac	1	34	590
Egg McMuffin	1	12	290
French fries	small	10	210
Kentucky Fried Chicken	breast	24	400
Pizza, cheese	1 slice large	10 – 13	250
Snacks, Treats			
Cookie, Chips Ahoy	1 (½ oz.)	2	50
Fig Newton	1 (½ oz.)	1	60
Brownie, from mix	1 small	5	140
Graham crackers	2 squares	1	60
Potato chips	1 oz. (about 18 chips)	9	150
Pretzels	1 oz.	1	110
Milky Way	1.75 oz. bar	8	220
M&Ms w/ peanuts	1.75 oz. bag	13	250
Reese's Peanut Butter Cups	2 (1.6 oz.)	15	280
Fruits and Vegetables			
Most varieties		negligible fat	

Oven Fries

Fast-food French fries can be a high-fat dietary disaster. But these oven fries are a popular alternative, even with children. They taste delicious and no one will complain the fries are low in fat.

Per person:

1   large baking potato

1   teaspoon oil, preferably olive or canola

Optional:

Your choice of: crushed red pepper, basil, garlic, oregano, salt, pepper

Preheat oven to 400°

1. Cut the potato lengthwise into 10 or 12 pieces. Place in a large bowl.

2. Add the oil and sprinkle with the seasonings. Toss to evenly coat.

3. Place on a nonstick baking sheet or a baking sheet treated with cooking spray.

4. Bake at 400° for 20 minutes. Turn the potatoes and continue to bake for another 10 to 15 minutes or until tender with golden-brown, crisp edges.

YIELD:	1 serving
Total calories:	260

	Grams	% of calories
CARB:	21	80
PRO:	4	5
FAT:	4	15

Oatmeal Cookies

Not only delicious, these cakey cookies are made with healthful canola oil and are a tasty way to spend a few grams of fat. Because they are easily digested, they are popular for a pre-exercise snack or a recovery food. This recipe makes about 5 dozen cookies—enough for a whole team of hungry marathoners!

1   cups milk

1   cup oil, preferably canola

2   eggs, or substitute

2   teaspoons vanilla extract

¾   cup sugar

1   cup firmly packed brown sugar

4   cups oatmeal

2   teaspoons baking soda

2   teaspoons salt

2   teaspoons cinnamon

1   cup raisins

3   cups flour, half white, half whole wheat, as desired

Preheat oven to 350°.

1. In a large bowl, beat together the milk, oil, eggs, and vanilla. Mix in the sugar and brown sugar. Add the oatmeal.

2. Blend in the baking soda, salt, cinnamon, and raisins. Fold in the flour.

3. Drop by teaspoons onto an ungreased baking sheet. Bake at 350° for 15 to 18 minutes.

YIELD:		about 60 cookies
Calories per recipe:		6,500
Calories per cookie:		110
	Grams	% of calories
CARB	16	60
PRO	2	10
FAT	4	30

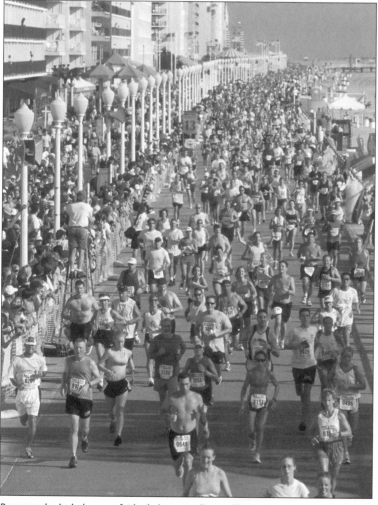

Runners who include some fat in their sports diet are likely to have greater endurance.
The fat is stored within muscles and provides the energy you need to get to the finish line.

CHAPTER 7

Water and Sports Drinks

WATER IS AN ESSENTIAL NUTRIENT EQUALLY IMPORTANT TO carbohydrates, proteins, and fats. Active people need adequate water for:

- *blood* to help carry oxygen and fuel to working muscles
- *urine* to help carry away the waste products
- *sweat* to dissipate heat
- *body fluids* to lubricate joints
- *gastric juices* to digest food.

Today's marathoners know that water is an important part of their training and racing diet, but that wasn't always the case. For example, in 1953, running regulations stated that marathoners could take water only after 9.3 miles. This contrasts to the twenty or more water stations provided along most of today's marathon courses!

All marathoners in all climates in all seasons should make the effort to replace sweat losses. This includes those who:

- race in the summer heat
- overdress for a winter training run
- sweat hard when working out on the health club's treadmill.

The American College of Sports Medicine recommends that you drink 4 to 8 ounces of fluid every 15 to 20 minutes of hard running. You should never allow yourself to become thirsty. That's a clear sign of dehydration. Dehydration slows you down, and in extreme cases, can contribute to medical problems.

Active people who replace fluid losses poorly during training and are chronically dehydrated tend to experience needless

COMPARING COMMON FLUID REPLACERS

Beverage (8 oz.)	Calories	Sodium (mg)	Potassium (mg)
Gatorade	50	110	30
Cola	100	5	—
Beer	100	12	60
Orange juice	110	2	475
Cranapple juice	175	5	70
Fruit yogurt	250	150	465
Possible losses in 2 hours	1,000	1,000	180

fatigue and lethargy. Don't let that happen to you! You can tell if you are well hydrated by monitoring your urine:

• You should urinate frequently (every 2 to 4 hours) throughout the day.

• The urine should be clear and of significant quantity.

• Your morning urine should *not* be dark and concentrated.

To determine how much you should drink during exercise, weigh yourself before and after an hour of training. If you have lost one pound (16 ounces) in one hour, you've lost one pint (16 ounces) of sweat, and should plan to drink accordingly during the next exercise session—at least 8 ounces every half-hour.

Strive to lose no more than 2 percent of your body weight per exercise session. That is, if you weigh 150 pounds, try not to lose more than 3 pounds of sweat during a workout.

Practice drinking fluids during training, so on marathon day you'll be familiar with the skills involved in drinking on the run as well as your body's capacity for fluids. If you plan to drink anything other than water (e.g., a sports drink), be sure that you have tried it during training as well.

● **SPORTS DRINKS**—Although water always has been and always will be a popular thirst quencher and fluid replacer, sports drinks are becoming more popular, particularly among

❝ *In the summer, before my long runs, I drive along the course and hide water bottles in the shrubs and behind telephone poles. Most of the time, the water is there when I run by and need a drink.* ❞

Amy Singer, Seattle, WA

● HOW MUCH SODIUM DO YOU LOSE IN SWEAT?

During an hour of running in the heat, you might lose 900 to 1,800 milligrams of sodium. The average male's body contains about 75,000 milligrams sodium (11 tablespoons of salt). The amount of sodium you lose in sweat depends upon:

How much salt you eat. The more salt you eat, the more salt you lose in sweat.

How much you exercise in the heat. If you are acclimatized to hot weather, you will conserve sodium to defend against sodium depletion. The sodium in one pound of sweat may be:

• 1,600 milligrams sodium for an unfit, unacclimatized person
• 1,200 milligrams for a fit but unacclimatized person
• 800 milligrams for a fit and acclimatized athlete.

You can easily replace the sodium losses by eating some of these popular recovery foods:

Food	Sodium (mg)	Food	Sodium (mg)
Pizza, ½ medium	1,400	Saltines, 10	400
Spaghetti sauce, 1 cup	1,200	Muffin, 1 medium	500
Soup, 1 cup	750	Salt, 1 packet	500

Although sports drinks are thought to be a sodium-rich recovery beverage, they are actually sodium poor, containing about 50 to 110 milligrams per 8 ounces.

endurance walkers and runners. During training sessions that last longer than 60 to 90 minutes, you'll perform better if you drink more than just plain water. That's where sports drinks come into the picture. They provide:

• small amounts of *carbohydrates* to fuel your mind and muscles
• *sodium* to enhance water absorption and retention
• *water* to replace sweat losses.

With the multitude of sports drinks on the market, it is easy to feel confused about what's best to drink and wonder which ones are better than the others. The bottom line is that you should choose the drink that you prefer; there are no significant advantages to one over the other.

The beverage perfect for all athletes in all events has yet to be designed. But in the quest for developing the ideal sports beverage, scientists have observed enormous individual differences among people's stomach function during exercise. This helps explain why some people choose plain water, others seek out a particular brand of sports drink, and some prefer to make their own concoction. The most important point is to *drink enough*. Any fluid, be it water or sports drink, is better than no fluid during extended exercise.

● **ELECTROLYTE REPLACEMENT**—When you sweat, you lose electrolytes such as sodium and potassium, two of the minerals that help maintain proper water balance in your tissues. Commercial sports drinks generally include these electrolytes. Although many marathoners believe the sodium and potassium are added to replace what is lost in sweat, these electrolytes are added primarily to increase the absorption rate of the water into your body.

Most runners don't have to worry about replacing electrolytes during exercise because the losses are generally too small to cause a deficit that will hurt performance and/or health. But, if you will be exercising for more than five hours, electrolyte losses can become problematic, particularly if you are drinking only water during that time. Your best bet during extended exercise is to drink sports drinks and eat foods that contain sodium and potassium.

● **HOW TO KEEP YOUR COOL**—The following true-false quiz is designed to test your knowledge about fluid replacement and help you survive the heat in good health and with high energy.

● *Drinking cold water during running will cool you off.*
True (but by a small margin). Although drinking cold water will cool you off slightly more than warmer water, the difference is small. That's because the water quickly warms to body temperature. The more important concern is quantity. Any fluid of any temperature is better than no fluid.

> ❝ **I've solved the problem of getting sticky from sports drinks that splash all over me when I'm running in a race: I cut a straw in half and tuck it under my watch-band. I then use the straw to drink from the cup while I'm running. I'm sure I end up drinking more fluids. The trick is to not drop the straw!** ❞
> Bill Franks, Sanbornton, NH

Despite popular belief, salt for athletes is not a four-letter word. The public health recommendations to reduce salt intake are directed to people who are overweight, underfit, and have high blood pressure—not lean, fit marathoners with low blood pressure.

How much salt do marathoners actually need?

- Salt (or more correctly *sodium*, the part of salt that is the health culprit) requirements depend upon how much you sweat. A "safe and adequate" sodium intake for the average person is 2,400 milligrams per day. The typical American intake is 3,000–6,000+ milligrams of sodium per day—this tends to cover the sodium needs of most marathoners.
- The rule of thumb is to add extra salt to your diet if you have lost more than four to six pounds of sweat (3–4 percent of your body weight pre- to post-exercise).
- Too little salt can result in fatigue, muscle cramps, and lack of thirst.
- Walkers and runners who sweat profusely day after day and eat primarily low-salt foods may benefit from adding a little sodium to replace that lost in sweat.

If I crave salt, should I eat it?

- Yes. Salt cravings signal that your body wants salt. If you hanker for some pretzels or salty foods, eat them!

- *Wetting yourself down during exercise with a cold sponge or towel will cool you off.*
  False. Surprising as it may seem, research suggests that sponging the face, arms, and trunk every 20 minutes with a cold towel does not reduce core body temperature. Psychologically, this cold towel may provide relief. Hence, your best bet is to drink often and sponge as desired, as long as you have enough fluids for both the inside and outside of your body.
- *Drinking water 30 minutes before exercise eliminates the need to drink fluids during a long training session.*
  False. Research suggests that drinking a quart of water before exercise is less effective than drinking an equal volume during exercise. Researchers aren't sure why, but they recommend the optimal approach: tank up beforehand *plus* drink enough to match your sweat losses during a long, strenuous run.

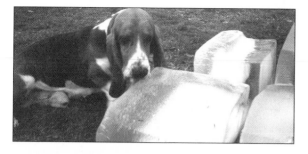

During the hot, dog days of summer, have plenty of cold fluids readily available. Cold beverages are more appealing than warmer ones, and you'll be apt to drink more, stay well-hydrated, and keep your cool.

- *Soda is a poor choice during exercise because the carbon dioxide in the bubbles will slow you down.*

  False. Historically, athletes were always warned to "de-fizz" carbonated beverages taken during exercise, fearing that the carbonation would interfere with oxygen transport and would also hurt performance. New studies comparing carbonated and non-carbonated soft drinks show bubbles will not hurt your performance nor result in stomach discomfort.

- *Don't bother to drink during a run that is shorter than an hour because the fluid has too little time to get into your system.*

  False. According to Larry Armstrong, exercise physiologist at the University of Connecticut, water can travel from stomach to skin in only 9 to 18 minutes after drinking. This water is essential for dissipating the 15 to 20 times more heat you produce during exercise as compared to that produced while you are at rest. Your safest bet is to try to match sweat losses with an equal volume of fluid during exercise.

- *Beer is an appropriate recovery fluid.*

  False. Although beer is a popular post-exercise recovery drink, its alcohol content has both a dehydrating and depressant effect. If you drink beer on an empty stomach (as commonly happens post-race), you can quickly negate the pleasurable "natural high" that you would otherwise enjoy. Wise beer-drinkers first have 1 to 2 glasses of water and eat some carbohydrate-rich foods (e.g., pretzels, pizza, crackers) and then they enjoy a beer or two in moderation.

> ❝ **In preparation for my long runs, I drink a lot of extra water the day before. I find this helps me feel better during the run and recover better afterwards. Getting up a few times during the night to go to the bathroom seems like a small price to pay!** ❞
>
> Amy Singer, Seattle, WA

Homemade Sports Drink

The main ingredients in commercial fluid replacers are:

Sugar. Sports drinks are 5 to 7 percent sugar; they contain about 12 grams of carbohydrate (50 calories) per 8 ounces—this is equal to 3 teaspoons of sugar per cup.

Sodium. They contain 50 to 110 milligrams of sodium per 8 ounces—this is equal to ⅛ teaspoon or 1 pinch of salt per cup.

This recipe comes close enough. Give it a try if you want a low-cost fluid replacer.

¼ cup sugar

¼ teaspoon salt

¼ cup orange juice

3½ cups cold water

1. In the bottom of a 1 quart bottle, dissolve the sugar in a little bit of hot water.
2. Add the salt and juice.
3. Add the cold water.
4. Quench that thirst!

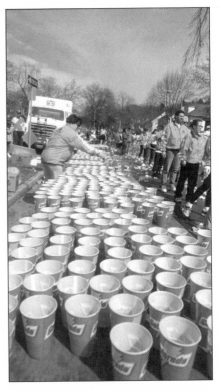

Sports drinks come in many flavors and brands. Find out which brand will be available on marathon day so you can test it during training.

YIELD:	1 quart or 4 (8-oz.) servings
Total calories:	200
Calories per serving:	50

	Grams	% of calories
CARB	12 gm	100
PRO	0 gm	0
FAT	0 gm	0
Sodium	110 mg	—
Potassium	30 mg	—

CHAPTER 8

Fueling Before You Exercise

JUST AS YOUR CAR WORKS BEST WITH GAS IN ITS TANK, YOUR BODY works best when it has been appropriately fueled. But food can sometimes be a problem for people who fear food-related upset stomachs that interfere with exercise. Running and fast walking jostles your stomach and enhances your risk of abdominal problems. An estimated 25 to 30 percent of runners may experience abdominal cramps, diarrhea, and/or the need for pit stops during or immediately after running.

Pre-exercise food promises advantages that can contribute to greater stamina and endurance. If you have always abstained from pre-exercise food based only on hearsay and habit, I encourage you to *try* a light snack. You might be pleasantly surprised by the benefits that come from fueling up rather than running on empty.

Because eating ability and food preferences vary in relation to the type and intensity of exercise and the time of day, all marathoners should *practice* pre-exercise eating. During training, you can learn through trial and error:

- what foods work best for your body
- when you should eat them
- what amounts are appropriate.

> **As a walker who became a runner, I have learned many things about my body. Initially, I couldn't eat before exercise or else I would get nauseated. Realizing I needed energy before heading out, I finally discovered that a glass of milk kick-starts me without ill effects. For longer distances, I bring dried fruit in my fanny pack.**
>
> Kim Holland, Maitland, FL

Any of the following recommendations regarding pre-exercise eating should be pondered and experimented with *during training*. You are an experiment of one; that is, only you can best determine what works best for you. And remember, food that you can tolerate on a normal training run may be intolerable during a race. Chalk that up to pre-event nervousness, not the food itself.

I emphasize *experiment during training* because here's what typically happens:

Marathoners read advertisements about special sports drinks, sports bars, supplements, or liquid meals. They are curious about trying these special products but because of their high price tag, they don't quite get around to buying them. Instead, they end up trying the free products provided by the sponsors on marathon day. In some instances they discover (much to their dismay) that for them the unfamiliar food causes an upset stomach, heartburn, diarrhea, or cramps. If they had sampled these new products during training, they would be confident about using or saving the race-day samples.

What (and whether) you eat before exercise will vary according to:

- *The type of exercise.* Pre-run food may make you uncomfortable, but pre-walk or pre-bike food might not cause any problems.
- *How hard you will be working.* You may be able to eat within ten minutes of an easy training run, an hour before a marathon, but need to wait three hours before a track workout.
- *How nervous you are.* Nothing will settle well if your stomach is in knots.

The general rule of thumb is that the harder you exercise the less likely you are to want to eat and the more likely you need to allow ample time between eating and exercising. Fast runners may feel nauseated at even the thought of pre-exercise food, but slow walkers will appreciate the added energy.

If you exercise at a pace that you can comfortably sustain for more than 30 minutes, you

> 66 I've found it's important to watch what I eat in the days preceding a long run or marathon, so I don't have to make extra stops along the way. For me, I find it best to limit certain vegetables and instead focus on pasta, rice, and breads. 99
>
> Jakson Badenhoop,
> Ponte Vedra Beach, FL

How much should you eat before you run? If you will be eating within an hour of running, exercise physiologist Mike Sherman recommends 0.5 gram carbohydrate per pound of body weight (or 1.0 gram carbohydrate per kilogram).

Body weight lbs. (kg)	Carbohydrates one hour pre-exercise	
	grams	calories
120 (55)	60	240
140 (64)	70	280
160 (73)	80	320
180 (82)	90	360

To translate this into food, choose from the following popular items:

Food	Carb (gm)	Calories
Bagel, 1 medium-large	60	320
Fruit yogurt, 1 cup	50	260
Fig Newtons, 4	44	240
Spaghetti, 1 cup cooked	40	200
Orange juice, 8 ounces.	25	110
Graham crackers, 4 squares	22	120
Oatmeal, ⅓ cup dry	20	110
Banana, 1 medium	25	105

can likely both exercise and digest food at the same time. At a training pace, the blood flow to your stomach is 60 to 70 percent of normal—adequate to maintain normal digestion processes.

If you are doing intense sprint work, your stomach essentially shuts down and gets only about 20 percent of its normal blood flow. This slows the digestion process so that any pre-exercise food will simply jostle along for the ride. It may feel uncomfortable and cause indigestion or heartburn.

" More marathons are won or lost in the portable toilets than they are on the roads. "
Bill Rodgers, Boston, MA

If you are in the experimental stage of developing your pre-exercise food plan for various intensity walks or runs, as well as for a marathon, the following information provides some helpful facts about the benefits of pre-exercise food. This information can help you on marathon day when the right combination of food and fluids will make or break your ability to complete the distance comfortably.

1. *Pre-exercise food helps prevent low blood sugar.* Why suffer with light-headedness, needless fatigue, blurred vision, and inability to concentrate when you can prevent these symptoms of hypoglycemia?

The carbohydrates in your pre-exercise snack are important because they fuel not only your muscles but also your mind. Adequate carbohydrates help you think clearly because your brain fuels itself with glucose, the sugar in your blood that is derived from carbohydrates. Successful athletes fuel both their muscles and their minds. As marathon legend Grete Waitz once commented, "Novice runners often fail to recognize how much mental energy and concentration is needed to run—especially to run a marathon."

Your blood sugar is maintained at a normal level by the release of sugar (glycogen) stored in your liver. If you have low blood sugar or a low liver glycogen, your brain will be left unfed. You will feel tired and you won't be able to concentrate on the task at hand. You may feel like you've "hit the wall." Why suffer when you can fuel yourself appropriately before you run?

If you run in the morning, you are likely to have to drag yourself through your workout if you haven't eaten anything between your 7:00 P.M. dinner and your 7:00 A.M. run. Similarly, if you choose to eat nothing between the pre-marathon pasta party and the 10:45 A.M. start of the New York City Marathon or the noon start of the Boston Marathon, you'll begin the event depleted and may end up devastated. Your blood sugar levels will have dropped, particularly if you tossed and turned all night with pre-race anxiety.

Some morning runners exercise with an

> **I've trained my body to thrive on pre-exercise food. From the beginning of my running career, I have always run with food in my stomach. I'd eat meals and snacks with my children so that I could enjoy family time with them, and then I'd run at night. I now have an iron stomach. I can eat and run—nothing bothers me.**
>
> Hal Gabriel, Newton, MA

● PRE-EXERCISE MEALS

To be sufficiently fueled for long training runs and walks, hard track workouts, shorter races, or the marathon, eat according to this schedule. *Always* drink additional fluids with and between meals to ensure complete hydration. If you are overly nervous, stressed, or have a sensitive stomach prior to the event, you may have to abstain from food on the day of competition. You should make a special effort to eat extra food the day before.

Morning events:
The day before: Minimal exercise
The night before: Eat a hearty, high-carbohydrate lunch, dinner, and bed-
                     time snack.
Race morning: Eat a light snack/breakfast to abate hunger feelings and
                     to replenish liver glycogen stores.

Afternoon events:
Day before: Minimal exercise
The night before: Eat a hearty high-carbohydrate dinner.
Race day: Eat a hearty high-carbohydrate breakfast and a light lunch.

Evening events:
Day before: Minimal exercise
               Eat high-carbohydrate meals.
Race day: Eat a hearty high-carbohydrate breakfast and lunch,
               followed by a light snack 1–3 hours prior to the event.

empty stomach and report that they have plenty of energy. They have likely eaten a substantial dinner and/or serious late-night snack to bolster liver glycogen stores and reduce their need for a morning energizer. This is not bad or wrong, as long as this pattern works well for them.

2. *Pre-exercise food helps settle the stomach, absorbs some of the gastric juices, and abates hunger feelings.* For many people, the stress associated with competition stimulates gastric secretions and contributes to an "acid stomach." Eating a small amount of food can help alleviate that problem.

The caloric density of a snack or meal affects the rate at which the food leaves your stomach. This explains why you can exercise comfortably soon after snacking on a few crackers or a piece of fruit but are better off waiting three or four hours after a heartier meal.

The general pre-exercise "rule of thumb" is to allow:

- 3–4 hours for a large meal to digest
- 2–3 hours for a smaller meal
- 1–2 hours for a blended or liquid meal
- less than an hour for a small snack, as tolerated

If you want to eat a full pre-marathon breakfast, simply allow ample time for it to digest by eating at 6:00 A.M.

66 **One year, the guy who was driving me to the marathon stopped for donuts, so I got some too. That was a mistake because I generally have only toast. The donuts landed like lead sinkers. I was in good shape for the marathon, but too many donuts did me in.** 99

Gerry Beagan, East Greenwich, RI

3. *Pre-exercise food fuels the muscles.* The food you eat even an hour before you exercise is digested into glucose and burned for energy. For example, one study showed that runners who ate 400 calories of sugar three hours before an easy four-hour run burned about 70 percent of the sugar. Without question, pre-run food that is well tolerated provides an energy boost that can enhance your stamina.

Historically, athletes were told to choose starchy complex carbohydrates, such as bagels, for the pre-race meal, in preference to sugary simple carbohydrates, such as soft drinks. The theory was that starches would contribute to a stable blood sugar level and sugary carbohydrates would contribute to a debilitating "sugar low" (hypoglycemic reaction). Today, we know that athletes should experiment with pre-run carbohydrates based on their *glycemic index*, that is, the food's ability to contribute glucose into the bloodstream (see page 71, *Glycemic Index of Some Common Foods*):

- Low glycemic foods (oatmeal, bran cereal) are desirable before a long run or walk because they provide sustained energy. They may reduce the need for consuming carbohydrates during endurance exercise to maintain normal blood sugar levels.
- High glycemic index foods (potatoes, rice) quickly elevate blood sugar. They can initiate hypoglycemic reactions in

The following list ranks foods according to their ability to elevate blood sugar given a 200 calorie (50 gram) dose of carbohydrates. Many factors influence this glycemic effect of a food, such as meal size, fiber content, other foods in the meal, and food preparation. Foods ranked higher than 70 are considered to have a high glycemic index.

Glucose	100	Banana	54
Potato, baked	85	Kidney beans, canned	52
Pretzels	81	Orange juice	52
Cheerios	74	Oatmeal	49
Bagel, white	72	Bread, multi-grain	48
Skittles	69	Peas, green	48
Soft drink, Fanta	68	Lentil soup	44
Raisins	64	Spaghetti	41
Table sugar	64	Orange	44
Honey	58	All-bran	42
Bran Chex	58	Snickers Bar	40
Bread, pita	57	Apple	38
Pizza	60	Yogurt, fruit	33
Corn, sweet	55	Milk, skim	32
Sweet Potato	54	Peanuts	15

Source: www.mendosa.com/gilists.htm

people sensitive to swings in blood sugar. Foods with a high glycemic index are preferable for recovery foods, when your depleted muscles readily absorb all available glucose.

Based on the latest research, you might want to experiment during training with your pre-run snack choices to determine if low glycemic foods bolster your performance. For example, if you have been eating a pre-exercise microwaved potato (a food with a high glycemic index), see if a bowl of lentil soup contributes to better performance (that is, unless the fiber causes problems with digestion).

4. *Pre-exercise beverages can provide fluids to fully hydrate your body as well as additional carbohydrates.* By tanking up on diluted juice or sports drinks before you exercise, you can help prevent dehydration as well as boost your carbohydrate and

energy intake. Whereas you are unlikely to starve during the marathon, you may become seriously injured due to dehydration. The best pre-exercise fluid choices include water, sports drinks, and diluted juices.

You should drink plenty of fluids not only before marathons and other races but also every day during training, in both hot weather and cold weather. You can confirm that you've had enough to drink by frequent urination and clear-colored urine. If your urine is dark and concentrated, you need more fluids. Refer to Chapter 7 for more information on hydration.

5. *Pre-exercise food can pacify your mind with the knowledge that your body is well fueled.* Before a long training run or walk, and particularly before a marathon, you don't want to waste any energy wondering if you've eaten enough. Appropriate eating can resolve that concern!

Pre-exercise food has great psychological value. If you firmly believe that a specific food or meal will enhance your performance, then it probably will. Your mind has a powerful effect on your body's ability to perform at its best. If you do have a "magic food" that assures athletic excellence, you should take special care to be sure this food or meal is available prior to the race.

- **FACTS ABOUT PRE-EXERCISE FOODS**—When experimenting with your pre-exercise foods, note the following information:
- *Liquid foods leave the stomach faster than solid foods.* If you have trouble with solid foods such as a bagel, you might want to experiment with liquids, such as juice or a canned liquid meal. One research study showed that a 450-calorie meal of steak, peas, and buttered bread took six hours to leave the stomach, whereas a blenderized variation of the same meal emptied from the stomach in four hours.
- *Carbohydrates are digested more easily than fatty foods.* Low-fat foods and meals (such as those listed in the sidebar, *High*

● HIGH-CARBOHYDRATE MEAL SUGGESTIONS

Some high-carbohydrate meal suggestions for both training and pre-marathon include tried-and-true foods such as:

Breakfast: cold cereals, oatmeal and other hot cereals, bagels, English muffins, pancakes, fruit, juice

Lunch: sandwiches (with the bread being the "meat " of the sandwich), fruit, hearty broth-based soups, thick-crust pizza

Dinner: pasta, potato, or rice entrées; veggies, breads, juice, fruit

Snacks: flavored yogurt, pretzels, crackers, fig bars, frozen yogurt, dry cereal, leftover pasta, zwieback, simple biscuit-type cookies, animal crackers, canned and fresh fruits, juice

Carbohydrate Meal Suggestions) tend to digest easily and settle well. In comparison, high-fat bacon-and-egg breakfasts, greasy hamburgers, tuna subs loaded with mayonnaise, and peanut butter sandwiches have been known to settle heavily and feel uncomfortable. Too much fat slows digestion, so the meal lingers longer in the stomach and may contribute to a weighed-down feeling.

A little fat, however, such as in a slice of cheese on toast, a teaspoon of peanut butter on a bagel, or the fat in some brands of sports bars, can be appropriate. It provides both sustained energy and satiety during long runs. Note that some marathoners can break all the sports nutrition rules and do well with even very high-fat foods. After all, steak-and-eggs was the pre-marathon breakfast of champions for many years!

- Pre-exercise sweets may cause a hypoglycemic reaction. Although most people can tolerate pre-exercise sweets without experiencing

> **❝ All the experimenting for marathon day should have been completed at least four weeks prior to the marathon. During these final four weeks, you should fine-tune what you've learned to be sure that your body can handle your choice of foods and fluids. ❞**
>
> John Correia, San Diego, CA
> Coach, Team in Training

negative effects on their performance, others are very sensitive to the swings in blood sugar that can occur after eating sugary foods. (Large doses of sugar can stimulate the secretion of large amounts of insulin to transport excessive

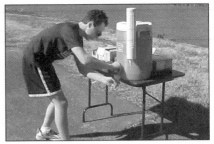

If you can't tolerate a pre-run snack, sports drinks during exercise will energize your run.

sugar out of the bloodstream. If too much sugar gets removed, you'll feel lightheaded and shaky.) If you are "sugar sensitive" and believe that sugar hurts your performance, refer back to the glycemic index information and take note of the low glycemic index foods that are least likely to cause blood sugar problems.

The best advice regarding pre-exercise sugar is for you to *avoid the need* for a sugar-fix by having appropriately timed meals prior to exercise. For example, if you crave sugar before an afternoon training run, know that you could have prevented the desire for quick-energy foods by having eaten a bigger breakfast and lunch. Skimping on those meals leaves you looking for a last-minute energizer that may hurt your performance.

Note that sugar taken *during* exercise does not contribute to a hypoglycemic reaction because muscles quickly use the sugar without the need for extra insulin.

● **SUMMARY**—Whether you are a walker or a runner, pre-exercise food will help you better enjoy your marathon training program. Just as you put gas in your car before you take it for a drive, you should put 100 to 300 calories of carbohydrate-rich food in your body before you exercise. Granted, each marathoner is an experiment of one, and some marathoners can tolerate food better than others; that's why you need to experiment during training to determine what pre-exercise menu works best for you.

> ❝ *I hate that feeling of being lightheaded and weak that I get after I eat sugary foods. I should know better than to eat sweets...my body just can't handle sugar unless it's after I've eaten a big meal.* ❞
>
> Marsha Jones, New York City

CHAPTER 9

Foods and Fluids During Long Walks and Runs

AS AN ENDURANCE ATHLETE, YOUR GOALS ARE TO prevent 1) dehydration and 2) hypoglycemia (low blood sugar). You can do this with fluids alone, or in combination with solid foods. Although elite runners are rarely seen consuming more than a sports drink, slower marathoners can thrive by consuming the proper intake of fluids and foods for their bodies.

During training and marathons, be sure to drink every 15 to 20 minutes. Remember, you want to *prevent* dehydration. Don't let yourself get thirsty. By drinking on a schedule—a target of 8 ounces, about 8 gulps, of water or sports drink every 15 minutes—you can minimize dehydration, maximize your performance, and reduce your recovery time.

Be sure to drink according to a schedule, not by how thirsty you are. And don't miss the early water stops; once you are dehydrated, you won't catch up. Losing only 2 percent of your body weight (3 pounds for a 150-pound person) from sweating hurts your performance and upsets your ability to regulate your body temperature. Refer to Chapter 7 for more details. To keep hydrated:

• If you are training with a group, take advantage

Beginning walkers need to carry with them food and fluids—energy bars, trail mix, sports drinks, even sandwiches and fruit—for any distance over 90 minutes. I've seen too many walkers dragging on the course, drained of energy and dehydrated. Many are walking for over 8 hours, and they would have normally eaten at least two meals during that time frame.

Becky Goodrum, Cleveland, OH

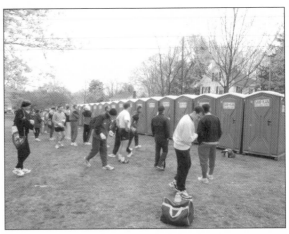

By experimenting with your food and fluid intake during training, you can minimize stomach upset—and visits to the toilet.

of the water stations your coach has set up along the route.

- If you are in a race, drink at every water station (or every 15 to 20 minutes).
- If you are training by yourself, set up your own water stops. This means planning a route that includes adequate water fountains, or driving the route before your run/walk and placing bottles filled with water or sports drinks in strategic locations.
- Take fluids with you. Some marathoners prefer to run with a Camelbak (water bladder that straps to the back) or other portable water system.

Drinking too much fluid to the point you feel the excess water sloshing around in your stomach can present a problem for some marathoners. The immediate solution is to stop drinking for a while. (Just as underhydrating can cause problems, so can overhydrating.) The long term solution is to practice drinking during training, so your body can adapt to the appropriate fluid intake.

You will feel better and perform better if you can replace not only water but also carbo-

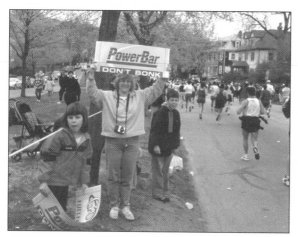
If you plan to eat energy bars during the marathon, also plan to drink plenty of water.

hydrates while running or walking. These carbohydrates help to maintain a normal blood sugar level as well as provide a source of energy for muscles. Then, during the marathon, when you come to the 18- or 20-mile mark, you can breeze right though it to the finish—and avoid "hitting the wall."

According to research, you might be able to increase your stamina by as much as 18 percent if you take in 0.5 grams of carbohydrate per pound of body weight (or 1 gram per kilogram) per hour of endurance exercise. For example, if you weigh 150 pounds, you should target about 75 grams of carbohydrates (300 calories) per hour. This could be:

- six 8-ounce glasses of a sports drink (50 calories per 8 ounces)
- four cups of sports drink and a banana
- two cups of sports drink plus a sports bar (plus extra water)
- five fig cookies plus water

This is more calories than many marathoners voluntarily consume during long runs or walks. Hence, you should have already practiced *programmed* eating and drinking. Then, on marathon day, you will know:

> ❝ *During a marathon, I prefer Swedish fish (gummy candy) over the gels because, as some runners know, gels sometimes send runners to the porta-potties during the race. Swedish fish give me an immediate sugar-fix, take the edge off the light-headed feeling, and don't leave me feeling sick afterwards. You can even bite down on this candy and it will stay in your teeth to keep the glucose coming. Perhaps this is not so great for your teeth, but it works for me.* ❞
>
> Valerie Watson, Cortland, OH

● POPULAR SNACKS DURING A LONG RUN

Solids:	Liquids:
Banana	Diluted, defizzed cola
Energy bars	Sports drinks
Bagel	Iced tea with honey
Tootsie Rolls	Diluted juice
Hard candies	Iced coffee with sugar
Chocolate Kisses	Go-Gurt (squeeze-pack yogurt)
Gummy candies	Gels
Vanilla cookies	Water (with solid food)

- what and how much you can tolerate
- how you can comfortably carry the fuel supply

Fanny packs or running shorts with multiple pockets are a good way to carry your snacks. You might also want to have friends replenish your supplies by meeting you at designated areas along the course. Think ahead and make a clear plan *before* marathon day. You must also be flexible. Who knows what happens when your body is pushed to the limit. Even tried-and-true favorites can become unpalatable.

Many marathoners prefer to consume carbohydrates by drinking some type of sugary fluid such as a sports drink, defizzed cola, or diluted juice. But solid foods can work well, too, as long as you drink plenty of water and can tolerate the food. Whereas the fastest runners are able to do well with just carbohydrate-containing *fluids*, slower runners and walkers, who are going to be on the marathon course longer, will likely do better with not only fluids but also *solids* that provide more calories. There is no magic to the special sports foods (e.g., gels, sports bars) that are available at your local running store. These engineered foods are simply pre-wrapped and convenient...but may also be expensive.

The carbs you consume during the marathon will also keep you in good spirits.

> 66 **For the walkers and slower runners who will be out for 6 or more hours, I recommend peanut-butter-and-honey sandwiches, just like mom made when you were a kid. Make them up the night before so the bread really soaks up the honey.** 99
>
> Earl Fenstremacher, Seattle, WA
> Coach, Joints in Motion

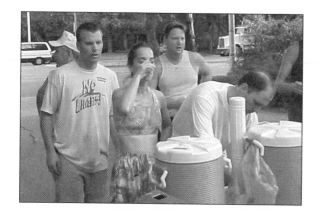

Drink sports drinks to prevent dehydration and to maintain a normal blood sugar, and you'll enjoy your long runs even more. These carbohydrate-containing fluids fuel both your muscles and your brain.

Some runners become moody, irritable, and irrational towards the end of a marathon. Running partners can become either the best of friends or the worst of enemies.

Many marathoners fear that fluids or foods taken during the event will cause diarrhea. Diarrhea commonly occurs in participants who lose more than 4 percent of their body weight during the race (6 pounds for a 150-pound person). Hence, the fluids you drink may actually help *prevent* diarrhea, not cause it.

I once talked to a runner who tried to abstain from drinking anything—even water—during a marathon in fear it would upset his stomach. He held off as long as he could without fluids. Then when he did succumb, he got diarrhea. Although he blamed the diarrhea on the drink, I tend to think the lack of prior fluid intake was the bigger problem.

● **SUMMARY**—Preventing dehydration and low blood sugar is crucial to a successful marathon. The fluids and foods that you consume during your long walks or runs should be an extension of your carbohydrate-rich daily training diet. Because each marathoner has individual tolerances and preferences, you should learn during

" *At about 18 miles into one marathon, I got into a huge argument with my running partner. He was tired, hypoglycemic, and feeling very irritable... he needed some carbohydrates to improve his spirits!* "

Jean Smith, Newton, MA

" *My running shorts have only a small key pocket, but I can stuff a couple of gel packs inside my bra. This works well for my long runs!* "

Amy Singer, Seattle, WA

training, through trial and error, what foods and fluids settle best and contribute to top competitive performance. Don't ruin months of physical training with poor nutrition training.

> **❝ Because I am a slow runner, I would typically get hungry during a long run and my energy level would plummet. I would try eating yet another sweet sports bar, which is full of carbohydrates, but it did very little to help; I had already had my fill of carbs. I realized that my body was craving something more solid; so I switched to a sports bar that has more protein. That has made all the difference. ❞**
>
> Brenda Van Oosten, Brecksville, OH

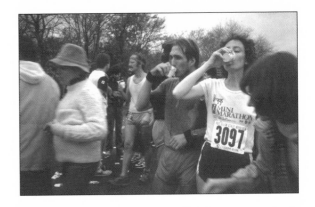

Knowing your sweat rate helps you know how much to drink at each water station. Consume at least 16 ounces of fluid for every pound of sweat you lose.

> **❝ I was given a lot of advice from lots of different kinds of runners, and I'm glad I took the time to figure out which advice works best for me. My long training runs were my marathon-rehearsals, during which I tried to figure out what worked and what didn't. By the time the marathon rolled around, I had a routine down that really worked for me. ❞**
>
> Amy Singer, Seattle, WA

CHAPTER 10

Recovery from Exhaustive Training

J UST AS FUELING BEFORE YOU EXERCISE IS IMPORTANT, SO IS REFUELING afterwards. Eating a proper recovery diet every day during training is very important if you are to endure repeated days— and months—of hard workouts. You may wonder if any special foods or fluids will hasten your recovery and help you feel better quickly. Here are the answers to questions athletes commonly ask about recovery foods.

● **WHAT IS THE BEST RECOVERY FOOD PLAN?**—To optimize the recovery process, you should eat 200 to 400 calories of carbohydrate-rich foods within two hours after the exercise bout, then repeat this every two hours for six hours. Good choices include apple juice, sweetened yogurts, soft drinks, potatoes, pasta, and, if you like the Bill Rodger's approach, a swig of maple syrup straight up!

Because you may have burned 1,000 calories or more during a 10 mile walk or run, sooner or later you'll be hungry and ready to eat. The replenishment process can take 24 to 48 hours and even longer if your muscles are damaged. If exercise initially kills your appetite or if even the thought of post-exercise food makes you nauseated, you can still drink the carbohydrates while you quench your thirst. With time, your hunger will return. For some people, this may not be until the next day.

> ❝ *When I come back from a long, hard training run, I'm generally exhausted and in need of some quick energy. I've been known to drink maple syrup right from the bottle. Tastes great!* ❞
>
> **Bill Rodgers, Boston, MA**

• **WHAT AND HOW MUCH SHOULD I DRINK?**—You should replace fluid losses as soon as possible to help your body restore normal water balance. Keep a water bottle (filled with water, juice, or sports drink) on your desk, in your car, or in your backpack, so you'll easily be able to drink enough to quench your thirst, and then drink some more. You may not feel thirsty, but your body may still need more fluids. Your goal is to have pale-colored urine in large volumes, then you'll know that you are well hydrated. Refer to Chapter 7 for more information.

Here are some fluid options:

- *Plain water.* It provides water but not the carbohydrates you need to replenish depleted muscle glycogen. Eat carbohydrate-rich foods with the water, such as a bagel, fruit, or pretzels. Eating some salty foods such as pretzels along with the plain water (or any beverage, for that matter) provides sodium which enhances fluid absorption and retention.

> **At the end of each long walk, I have found that I recover much more quickly if I sip on orange juice and eat at least half a banana.**
>
> Shelley Smith, Highlands Ranch, CO

- *Soft drinks.* Colas, in particular, are popular recovery fluids. Granted, soft drinks lack nutritional value and are filled with empty calories, but they do offer both carbohydrates and fluids. Most colas also offer caffeine, which for some may provide welcome stimulation. Historically, marathoners have been told to avoid caffeine, which, because of its diuretic effect, was believed to hamper their efforts to replace fluids. Recent research suggests that the diuretic effect is insignificant and is unlikely to have any detrimental effect on recovery.

- *Juices.* Fruit and vegetable juices are always an excellent choice because they not only offer a rich supply of carbohydrates, they also offer the vitamin C your body needs to optimize healing.

- *Sports drinks.* Commercial fluid replacers that are designed to be taken during exercise are dilute and provide fewer recovery carbohydrates than juices or soft drinks. In 16 ounces of cranapple juice you can get the same amount of carbohydrates as in 48 ounces of a commercial fluid replacer.

Your muscles are most receptive to replacing depleted glycogen stores immediately after exercise. For optimal recovery, target approximately 0.5 gram
of carbohydrate per pound of body weight (or 1 gram carbohydrate per
kilogram) every two hours for six hours following exercise.

Carbohydrates for recovery:

Body weight lbs (kg)	Carbohydrate grams	calories
120 (55)	60	240
140 (64)	70	280
160 (73)	80	320
180 (82)	90	360

If you can't tolerate solid foods immediately following a hard run or marathon,
simply drink carbohydrate-rich fluids and/or eat watery foods, having mini-
meals or snacks every two hours.

Some popular choices include:

Food	Amount	Carb. (grams)	Total calories
Gatorade	1 cup	12	50
Apple juice	1 cup	30	120
Cranapple juice	1 cup	45	180
Cola	12 oz. can	38	150
Banana	1 large	35	150
Fruit yogurt	1 cup	40	240
PowerBar	1	45	230
Baked potato	1 large	50	220

- *Commercial recovery drinks.* These high-carbohydrate beverages are sweetened with a type of sugar that tastes less
sweet, so it is more palatable in high concentrations. They
are convenient, but they offer nothing that cannot be found
in standard foods.

● **DO I NEED EXTRA SALT TO REPLACE WHAT I LOSE IN SWEAT?—**
In most cases, marathoners can replace more than enough salt
by eating standard foods after exercise. Both walkers and runners lose some sodium (a part of salt) in sweat but are unlikely to deplete their body stores, even during a marathon. As I

● REPLACING POTASSIUM LOSSES

During an hour of running in the heat, you might lose 100 to 400 milligrams of potassium. To replace this, you can eat some of these popular recovery foods.

Food	Amount	Potassium (mg)
Potato	1 large baked	800
Banana	1 medium	450
Orange juice	1 cup	430
Yogurt	1 cup plain	350
Raisins	¼ cup	300

Sports drinks are potassium-poor choices, having about 25 to 45 milligrams per 8 ounces. Juices, fruits, and vegetables tend to be the better choices for potassium.

> **My favorite recovery foods are a handful of salted, dry-roasted peanuts and a stack of Fig Newtons.**
>
> Earl Fernstermacher, Seattle, WA

mentioned in Chapter 7, during three hours of sweaty exercise, you might lose about 1,800 to 5,600 milligrams of sodium. Since the average 150-pound person's body contains about 97,000 milligrams of sodium, this 2 to 6 percent loss is relatively insignificant.

Athletes who may need extra salt include those who train in cold weather yet run a marathon in warm weather. This sometimes happens, for example, with Boston Marathoners if they train throughout the winter but compete on what turns out to be an unusually warm spring day. It also happens with people who live in cold climates, like Minnesota, but run a marathon where the weather is hot, such as Hawaii. Note that slower marathoners who exercise continuously for more than four to six hours are more likely to need a little extra salt than faster marathoners.

If you crave salt, you should respond appropriately by eating salty, carbohydrate-rich foods such as salted pretzels, soups, crackers and/or baked potatoes sprinkled with salt.

● **DO I NEED EXTRA POTASSIUM?**—Probably not. Like sodium, you lose some potassium when you sweat, but you are unlikely to deplete your body stores. During three hours of exercise, you might lose 300 to 1,200 milligrams of potassium (.001 to .007 percent of your body stores). The typical American diet provides 4,000 to 7,000 milligrams of potassium and can easily replace that lost in sweat, particularly if you eat potassium-rich foods, such as fruits and vegetables.

● **DO I NEED EXTRA PROTEIN?**—You do not need to "protein load" and eat a protein-rich recovery diet. Eating too much meat and other protein foods leaves you eating less of the carbohydrate-rich foods that you need to refuel depleted glycogen stores. Marathoners can meet their protein needs by eating protein as part of a balanced training diet. Eating a serving of protein-rich food at two meals (such as turkey on sandwich at lunch and lean hamburger in spaghetti sauce at dinner) and eating three servings of dairy foods (such as low-fat milk, yogurt, or cheese) each day gives most marathoners enough protein to build and repair muscle. Refer to Chapter 5 for more information.

Many marathoners report craving protein after hard exercise. If that's the case for you, eat the protein, but be sure to also eat carbohydrate-rich foods as an accompaniment (a bagel with eggs, hearty bread with peanut butter, potato and rolls with steak). This balance will help you rebuild and refuel, as well as enjoy the process.

● **RECOVERING FROM THE MARATHON**—Congratulations! Your most important job post-marathon is to relax, enjoy yourself, and be proud of your accomplishment. Indulge with lots of water, carbohydrates, even tasty reward foods. Because you'll have plenty of time after the marathon to replace depleted glycogen stores, you can be less strict with choosing recovery carbohydrates (as discussed at the beginning of this chapter) and go with what you crave. If you celebrate with beer, wine, or Champagne, be sure to eat first so that you are not drinking alcohol on an empty stomach, and also have some juice or soft drink to supply your muscles with water and carbohydrates. Allow yourself to rest, heal, and eat well. And if your legs and feet will allow, you might even enjoy the post-marathon dance party.

Yes, you do want to continue to eat:

- plenty of post-marathon recovery carbohydrates to refuel your muscles
- adequate protein (to help with healing damaged muscles)
- potassium-rich fruits and juices and salty foods to replace electrolyte losses.

But you need not be obsessive with your recovery diet because you will not be demanding much from your muscles for a while. A nice massage and a gentle swim or bike ride to loosen stiff muscles without pounding the joints are good ideas. The standard practice is to allow an easy day for every mile run—that's almost a month of gentle exercise.

● RECOVERY RECIPES

Chocolate Lush

This brownie pudding is a tasty treat and a welcome reward for tired marathoners who want a carbohy-drate-rich, low-fat dessert. It forms its own sauce during baking and, of course, tastes even better when topped with (low-fat) ice cream!

1   cup flour

¾   cup sugar

2   tablespoons unsweetened cocoa powder

2   teaspoons baking powder

1   teaspoon salt

½   cup milk

2   tablespoons oil, preferably canola

2   teaspoons vanilla extract

Topping:

¾   cup firmly packed brown sugar

¼   cup unsweetened cocoa powder

1¾ cups hot water

Preheat oven to 350°.

1. Treat an 8-inch square baking pan with cooking spray.

2. In a medium bowl, stir together the first five ingredients (flour through salt). Add the milk, oil, and vanilla. Stir until smooth.

3. Pour the batter into the prepared pan.

4. For the topping, In a separate bowl, combine the brown sugar, cocoa, and hot water. Pour this mixture on top of the batter in the pan.

5. Bake at 350° for 40 minutes, or until lightly browned and bubbly.

YIELD:	9 servings
Total calories:	2,100
Calories per serving:	230

	Grams	% of calories
CARB	46	80
PRO	3	5
FAT	4	15

Chicken Black Bean Soup

This soup is an excellent recovery food. It offers fluid, sodium, carbohydrates, protein, and vitamins—everything your body needs to rebuild and refuel. Plus, the soup can be made in advance, so it will be ready and waiting for your arrival after a long run.

4 chicken breast halves, skinned and boned

5 cups broth or water

2 carrots, peeled and sliced

2 tomatoes, chopped

½ onion, chopped

3 to 5   cloves garlic, crushed

2 16-ounce cans black beans, rinsed and drained

1 teaspoon dried oregano

Salt and pepper to taste

Optional:

2 to 4   cups cooked pasta, shells or bow-ties

2 ounces (½ cup) grated Cheddar cheese

½ cup marsala wine

Hot red pepper flakes

Place all of the ingredients (except the optional ingredients) in a large stock pot. Bring to a boil, reduce the heat, and simmer for about 20 minutes or until the chicken is done.

1. Remove the chicken from the broth and set it aside to cool. Keep the broth over low heat.

2. Dice the chicken into small pieces and return it to the soup. Add the cooked pasta and marsala wine, if desired. Heat the soup through.

3. Garnish with grated cheese and red pepper flakes, if desired.

YIELD:	4 servings
Total calories:	1,200
Calories per serving:	300

	Grams	% of calories
CARB	33	45
PRO	34	45
FAT	3	10

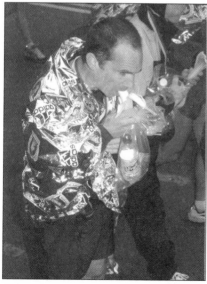

To facilitate a speedy recovery, eat as soon as tolerable post-marathon.

CHAPTER 11

Marathon Week: Nutrition Preparations

BECAUSE 26.2 MILES IS A VERY LONG DISTANCE TO WALK OR RUN, YOU want to be sure to fuel your muscles optimally with carbohydrates. This can make a *big* difference in your marathon enjoyment. Carbohydrate-loading, however, means more than just eating a pile of pasta. Here's some food for thought.

● **PRE-MARATHON TRAINING DIET**—You can't simply eat a big dinner of pasta the night before the marathon and expect to run well. Your muscles have to be trained to store carbohydrates, and that naturally happens as a part of a daily walking or running program.

To support the rigors of marathon training, you need to eat a carbohydrate-rich sports diet *every* day as the foundation for *every* meal. Runners and walkers who carbo-load every day (i.e., eat a diet with 55 to 65 percent of the calories from carbohydrates):

● can train better because their muscles are better fueled
● can continue eating the same foods pre-marathon.

The last thing you want to do is change your diet before the marathon.

To avoid nutritional mistakes on marathon day, during training you should:

● Practice eating your planned pre-marathon breakfast. If you will be traveling a long distance to the marathon, be sure this tried-and-true food will be available on marathon day.
● Start your long training runs and walks at the time you'll be running or walking on marathon day. For example, the

● PASTA

Pasta comes in at least 26 shapes, ranging from plain spaghetti strands to bowties. All the shapes are made from the same wheat-and-water dough, sometimes tinted with vegetable juice (e.g. spinach, tomato). The best pasta is made from durum wheat that has been ground into fine granules called semolina or into durum flour. Durum wheat has a high gluten (protein) content, which gives the pasta a firm texture. Whole-wheat pasta, in comparison, tends to have more fiber and be softer; soy pastas are even softer.

When trying to decide which shape of pasta to use for a meal, the rule of thumb is to use twisted and curved shapes (such as twists and shells) with meaty, beany, and chunky sauces. The shape will trap more sauce than would the straight strands of spaghetti or linguini.

Although pasta is an international favorite food of runners, you may struggle with understanding which shape is named what. Here is the translation into English for runners who are not fluent in pasta:

Name	Shape
Capelli d'angelo	Angel's hair
Conchiglie	Shells
Conchigliette	Little shells
Farfalle	Butterflies (or bowties)
Fusilli	Twisted spaghetti strands
Fettuccini	Flat, wide spaghetti
Linguini	Flat, thin spaghetti
Manicotti	Big tubes
Penne	Skinny tubes with pointed ends
Rigatoni	Tubes
Rotelle	Twists
Route	Cart wheels
Stelline	Little stars
Vermicelli	Very thin spaghetti
Ziti	Small tubes

The quickest cooking pastas include angel hair, alphabets, and the little stars, stelline. The time consuming part is waiting for the water to boil. If desired, you can cook the pasta in half the amount of water and it will cook okay in less time.

● HOW TO COOK PASTA

The perfect boiled pasta is tender, yet firm to the teeth—"al dente" as the Italians say. To cook pasta perfectly, follow these rules:

- Use a big pot filled with water, so the individual pieces of pasta can float freely. Allow 10 minutes for the water to reach a rolling boil.

- Allow 4 quarts of water per pound of dry pasta. Plan to cook no more than 2 pounds of pasta at a time; otherwise, you may end up with a gummy mess.

- To keep the water from boiling over, add 1 tablespoon of oil to the cooking water. You can also add 1 to 2 tablespoons of salt if desired to heighten the flavor of the pasta.

- Bring the water to a vigorous, rolling boil before you add the pasta. Then, add the pasta in small amounts that will not cool the water too much and cause the pieces to clump. When cooking spaghetti or lasagna, push down the stiff strands as they soften, using a long-handled spoon

- If the water stops boiling, cover the pot, turn up the heat, and bring the water to a boil again as soon as possible.

- Cooking time will depend on the shape of the pasta. Pasta is done when it starts to look opaque. To tell if it is done, lift a piece of pasta (with a fork) from the boiling water, let it cool briefly, then carefully pinch or bite it (being sure not to burn yourself). The pasta should feel flexible but still firm inside.

- When done, drain the pasta into a large colander set in the sink, using potholders to protect your hands from the steam. Shake briefly to remove excess water, then return it to the cooking pot or to a warmed serving bowl.

- To prevent the pasta from sticking together as it cools, toss the pasta with a little olive or canola oil or tomato sauce.

Boston Marathon starts at noon, so do some training runs at noon. The Disney Marathon in Orlando starts at 6:00 A.M., so do some early morning runs.
- Learn how much pre-exercise food you can eat and then still run or walk comfortably.
- Practice drinking the sports drink that will be available on race day as well as any mid-run foods you plan to eat.

This will help reduce surprises!

• **THE WEEK BEFORE THE MARATHON**—The biggest change in your schedule during the week before your marathon should be in your *training*, not in your food. You'll want to taper off your training so that your muscles have the opportunity to become fully fueled. Don't bother with any last-minute hard training that will burn off carbohydrates rather than allow them to be stored. Instead, for a Sunday marathon, limit yourself to four miles on Monday and Tuesday, rest on Wednesday, three miles on Thursday, rest on Friday (travel day) and Saturday (light sightseeing).

You need not eat hundreds more calories this week. You simply need to exercise less. This way, the 600 to 1,000 calories you generally expend during training can be stored as fuel in your muscles. All during this week, you should maintain your tried-and-true, high-carbohydrate training diet. Drastic changes commonly lead to upset stomachs, diarrhea, or constipation. For example, carbo-loading on an unusually high amount of fruits and juices might cause diarrhea. Too many white-flour, low-fiber bagels, breads, and pasta might clog your system.

Be sure that you are *carbo*-loading, not *fat*-loading. Some runners eat two pats of butter per dinner roll, big dollops of sour cream on a potato, and enough dressing to drown a salad. These fatty foods fill the stomach and the fat cells but leave the muscles less fueled. Your best bet is to trade the extra fats for extra carbohydrates:

- Instead of having one roll with butter for 200 calories, have two plain rolls for 200 calories.
- Have pasta with tomato sauce or low-fat sauces rather than oil-based or cheese-based toppings.
- Enjoy low-fat frozen yogurt instead of gourmet ice cream.

Many marathoners totally avoid protein-rich foods the days before the marathon. This is

> " *During one of our training meetings, we prepare an "energy food buffet." The other coach and I bring a variety of energy bars, gels, and sports drinks. We cut, squirt, and pour so that our marathoners can taste a variety of flavors and textures. By having our buffet, people can sample a wide variety of products. They can then purchase what they think might work for them and try those on their training runs. We constantly remind them: Don't use it in the race if you haven't trained with it!* "
>
> Chris Davis, Duluth, MN
> Coach, Joints in Motion

The following quick and easy pasta toppings are a change of pace from the standard tomato sauce straight from the jar. Try them *before* marathon week!

- Steamed, chopped broccoli
- Salsa
- Salsa heated in the microwave, then mixed with cottage cheese
- Olive oil with red pepper flakes
- Low-fat Italian salad dressing mixed with a little Dijon mustard
- Low-fat or fat-free salad dressings of your choice with steamed vegetables
- Low-fat or fat-free sour cream and Italian seasonings
- Chili with kidney beans (and cheese)
- Parmesan cheese and a sprinkling of herbs (basil, oregano, Italian seasonings)
- Chicken breast sautéed with oil, garlic, onion, and basil
- Lentil soup (thick)
- Spaghetti sauce with a spoonful of grape jelly (adds a "sweet 'n sour" taste)
- Spaghetti sauce with added protein: canned chicken or tuna, tofu cubes, canned beans, cottage cheese, ground beef or turkey

unnecessary because your body still needs protein on a daily basis. Also, endurance runners even burn a little protein for energy. Hence, you can and should eat a small serving of low-fat proteins such as poached eggs, yogurt, turkey, or chicken as the accompaniment to the meal (not the main focus), or plant proteins such as beans and lentils (as your intestines can tolerate them).

> 66 *I never eat a very big meal the night before a marathon, as it usually gives me trouble the next day. I prefer to eat a bigger lunch, then a lighter supper.* 99
>
> Grete Waitz, Norway

● **THE DAY BEFORE THE MARATHON**—By now, you may have gained about three to four pounds, but don't panic. This weight gain reflects water weight. For every ounce of carbohydrate stored in your body (i.e., glycogen), you store about three ounces of water. You can tell if your muscles are well saturated with carbohydrates if the scale has gone up two or three pounds.

Instead of relying upon a huge pasta dinner the night before the marathon, you might want to enjoy a substantial carbo-feast at breakfast or lunch. This earlier meal allows plenty of time for

● RICE FOR RUNNERS

Not all marathoners carbo-load on pasta. Rice is a fine alternative, preferably brown rice. Brown rice retains the fiber-rich bran, which is removed during the refining process to make white rice.

Cooking Tips:

- Because of its tough bran coat and germ, brown rice needs about 45 to 50 minutes to cook; white rice only about 20 to 30 minutes.
- Consider cooking rice in the morning while you are getting ready for work, so that it will be waiting to be simply reheated when you get home.
- When cooking rice cook double amounts to have leftovers that you can either freeze or refrigerate.

Portions:

- 1 cup raw white rice = 3 cups cooked = 700 calories
- 1 cup raw brown rice = 3 to 4 cups cooked = 700 calories

Rice is popularly cooked by two methods:

1. Bring a saucepan of water to a full boil.
2. Stir in ⅓ to ½ cup of rice per person plus 1 to 2 teaspoons salt, as desired.
3. Simmer about 20 minutes, or until a grain of rice is tender when you bite into it. (For brown rice, simmer for 50 minutes.)
4. Drain into a colander, rinse it under hot tap water to remove the sticky starch, and put it back into the saucepan.
5. Keep the rice warm over low heat, fluffing it with a fork.

OR

1. For each one cup of rice, put two cups of water into a saucepan, and a teaspoon salt, as desired.
2. Bring to a boil, then cover and turn the heat down low.
3. Let the rice cook undisturbed until it is tender and all the water has been absorbed.
4. Stir gently with a fork. Do not over-stir, which may result in a gluey mess.
5. This method retains more of the vitamins that otherwise get lost into the cooking water.

the food to move through your system. Or, eat at both times!

You'll be better off eating a little bit too much than too little on the eve of the marathon. But you don't want to *over*eat either. Learning the right balance takes practice. Let each preparatory race and long run be opportunities to learn.

Be sure to drink extra water, juices, and even carbohydrate-rich soft drinks, if desired. Abstain from too much wine, beer, and other alcoholic beverages because they can have a dehydrating effect. You want to be well saturated with water, not flushing needed fluids down the toilet.

● MARATHON MORNING—With luck, you'll wake up to a clear, crisp day that makes you want to jump out of bed and walk or run! Before embarking upon your day's task, be sure to eat breakfast. One of the biggest nutritional mistakes made by novice marathoners is eating too little beforehand, fearing that eating will result in an upset stomach.

As I've repeatedly mentioned, be sure to eat pre-marathon foods that are tried-and-true. That is, don't feast on a pancake breakfast marathon morning only to discover that pancakes settle like a lead balloon. Some marathoners can eat a bagel, juice, or a light breakfast one to three hours before the event; many carry familiar

> 66 **There's more to preparing for the marathon than just eating carbs. The marathon is a mind game. You have to program your mind in order to do it.** 99
>
> Hal Gabriel, Newton, MA

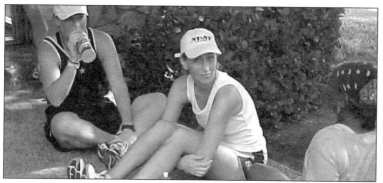

While waiting for the marathon to start, think positively. Trust that your body is well-fueled, well-trained, and ready to perform at its best.

foods with them to the start. Others want six hours for their stomach to empty; they've learned they run best if they wake up at 4 A.M., eat a bowl of oatmeal, and then go back to bed.

Drink plenty of fluids on marathon morning. Water and sports drinks are popular choices. Some runners drink coffee for stimulation or for its laxative effect. Others prefer to abstain because they are already nervous and jittery and have no need for an added buzz. Choose what's best for your body—do what you normally do before your long training runs.

Whatever beverage you like to drink, take it with you in a throw-away bottle so you'll have it available at the race. Because water takes about 45 to 90 minutes to move through your system, you can drink several glasses up to two hours before the marathon, have time to urinate the excess, then tank up again 5 to 15 minutes before the starting gun. With pre-race nerves, don't be surprised if you are urinating twenty times!

● **FUELING DURING THE MARATHON**—Your job during the marathon is to prevent dehydration and to maintain a normal blood sugar level. I have discussed those topics in chapters 7, 8, 9, and 10. Remember, you should be doing noth-

> ❝ *The first marathon I ran started at 11:00 A.M. The friend who talked me into it told me not to eat beforehand. Not knowing any better, I followed his advice. We got up at 5:30 and by the time we got to the start area, I was starved. I found half a donut on the ground, and in desperation, I ate it. I was hungry all morning, and by the time I finished the marathon I was starved.* ❞
>
> Pam Duckworth,
> Steamboat Springs, CO

ing new, special, or different during the marathon. Stick with what has worked for you in your training runs. That is, stick with the tried-and-true.

● **SUMMARY**—By marathon day, you should be well trained: You should have not only strong muscles but also a strong knowledge of the foods and fluids you need to fuel those muscles. Knowing you are nutritionally prepared, you need not fear that you will tire prematurely, or "hit the wall." Instead, you can focus on the day's job—enjoying the 26.2 miles with energy to spare!

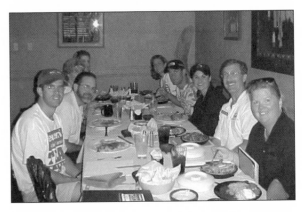

Sharing an enjoyable pre-marathon dinner adds to your marathon memories.

CHAPTER 12

Tips for the Traveling Marathoner

IF YOU ARE ONE OF THE MANY MARATHONERS WHO WILL BE TRAVELing to a fun-filled location to participate in a marathon, be sure to fight the urge to do too much exploring. Better yet, save the sightseeing until *after* the marathon. Fully fuel your muscles by putting your feet up and resting your legs. Relax with some juices and other tried-and-true carbohydrates, and visualize yourself completing the entire distance smoothly, strongly, and successfully.

Traveling marathoners are confronted with nutritional challenges, including:

- finding their familiar sports foods pre-marathon
- avoiding the rich temptations that lurk in every restaurant, deli, and push cart.

All too often when traveling, you can get sidetracked by the confusion and excitement of being in a new city.

One key to successfully selecting a top-notch sports diet when you are traveling is to bring some foods with you. This is not foolproof, however. For example, elite marathoner Gelindo Bordin of Italy (known as a food-lover extraordinaire) schlepped not only his own pasta and grateable hard cheese to New York for the marathon, but also a small hot plate on

> **❝ When I would travel to marathons, I'd eat the pasta dinner, then go back to the hotel room, where I'd relax on the bed, watch TV, and carbo-load on a stack of Fig Newton's and a quart of orange juice. Not everyone can handle that many Fig Newton's, but they sure worked for me and helped give me my best times! ❞**
>
> Gerry Beagan, E. Greenwich, RI

> **Plan on bringing what you need to the marathon. Do not assume the event will supply you with what you are accustomed to eating. You have spent six months preparing for this marathon; do not jeopardize your ability to enjoy it by eating some unfamiliar food.**
>
> Matt Keil, San Jose, CA
> Coach, Team in Training

which to cook in his hotel. The only problem was that the water was different in New York City. To his dismay, this not only affected his cooking but also negated his beloved espresso.

The 1992 New York City Marathon winner Willie Mtolo of South Africa also brought a hot plate to cook his traditional pre-marathon food: phutu, a cornmeal-based porridge. His cooking, however, promptly set off the hotel's fire detectors. Mtolo and his fiancée used towels to fan the smoke out the windows, waited for the firefighters to leave, then finished their meal in peace. Such can be the price of eating your familiar foods in preparation for the marathon!

To help you better accommodate a high-carbohydrate sports diet into your traveling routine, here are a few tips.

Breakfast:

- At a restaurant or deli, order pancakes, French toast, whole-wheat toast, or English, bran, or corn muffins. Add jelly, jam, or maple syrup for extra carbohydrates, but hold the butter or request that it be served on the side so that you can better control the amount of fat in your meal.
- Order a large orange juice or tomato juice. This can help compensate for a potential lack of fruits or veggies in the other meals.
- For a hotel stay, you might want to save time and money by packing your own cereal, raisins, and spoon. Either bring powdered milk or buy a half-pint of low-fat milk at a local convenience store. A water glass or milk carton can double as a cereal bowl.

Lunch:

- Find a deli or restaurant that offers wholesome breads. Request a sandwich that emphasizes the bread, rather than the filling (preferably lean beef, turkey, ham, or chicken). Hold the mayonnaise, and instead, add moistness with mustard or ketchup, sliced tomatoes, and lettuce. Add more carbohydrates with juice, fruit, fig bars (brought from a corner store), or yogurt for dessert.

- At fast-food restaurants, the burgers, fried fish, special sandwiches, and French fries have a very high fat content. You'll get more carbohydrates by sticking to the spaghetti, baked potatoes, chili, or thick-crust pizza selections.
- Request thick-crust pizza (with veggie toppings) rather than thin-crust pizza with pepperoni or sausage.
- At a salad bar, generously pile on the chickpeas, three-bean salad, beets, and fat-free croutons. Take plenty of bread. But don't fat-load on large amounts of butter, salad dressings, and mayonnaise-smothered pasta and potato salads.
- Baked potatoes are a super choice if you request them plain rather than drenched with butter, sour cream, and cheese toppings. For moistness, try mashing the potato with milk (usually by special request) rather than butter, or eat them with ketchup.
- Hearty soups (such as split pea, minestrone, lentil, vegetable, or noodle) accompanied by crackers, bread, a plain bagel, or an English muffin provide a satisfying, carbohydrate-rich, low-fat meal.
- Both juices and soft drinks are rich in carbohydrates. Juices, however, are nutritionally preferable for vitamin C, potassium, and wholesome goodness.

Dinner:
- If possible, check out the restaurant beforehand to make sure that it offers wholesome carbohydrates (pasta, baked potatoes, rice, steamed vegetables, salad bars, homemade breads, fruit, juice), broiled foods, and low-fat options. To be on the safe side, save the exotic restaurants for after the marathon! Inquire how dishes are made. Request they be prepared with minimal fat.
- Eat the breads and rolls either plain or with jelly. Replace the butter calories with high-carbohydrate choices: another slice of bread, a second potato, soup and crackers, juice, sherbet, or frozen yogurt.
- When ordering salads, always request the dressing be served on the side. Otherwise, you may get as many as 400 calories

of oil or mayonnaise—fatty foods that fill your stomach but leave your muscles unfueled.

Snacks and munchies:
- Pack your own snacks. Some suggestions include: whole-grain bagels, muffins, rolls, crackers, pretzels, energy bars, fig bars, oatmeal-raisin cookies, granola, oranges, raisins, dried or fresh fruit, and juice boxes.
- Buy wholesome snacks at a convenience store: small packets of trail mix, bananas, dried fruit, yogurt, V-8 juice or fruit juice, bagel, hot pretzel, slice of thick-crust pizza, small sandwich, or cup of soup.

● **SUMMARY**—Traveling is fun but temptation-filled. Do your best to stick to tried-and-true foods that you know will settle well and not upset your digestive system. Save the food experimenting until after the marathon. If you have any doubts about the availability of familiar foods, plan ahead and bring some "safe" foods with you.

●TRAVELER RECIPE

Breakfast for Travelers

If you're heading for a race out of town, this breakfast is portable, easy, and substantial. You can mix and match your own combinations of fruits and cereals.

In a plastic container with a lid, combine:

½ cup raw oatmeal

½ cup Grape-Nuts cereal or other cereal

¼ cup raisins or other dried fruit

½ cup dry non-fat milk powder

When you are ready to eat, simply add 1 cup of cold water and shake!

YIELD:		1 serving
Calories per serving:		700

	Grams	% of calories
CARB	135	75
PRO	35	20
FAT	3	5

CHAPTER 13

Calculating Your Calorie Needs

AS A MARATHONER, YOU ARE CONSTANTLY BURNING CALORIES. IF you think of your calorie needs in terms of an accounting system, you can maintain a high level of energy throughout the day by depositing calories *regularly* into your calorie account. If you know how many calories your body requires, you can take the necessary steps to:

- maintain an even flow of energy all day long
- appropriately fuel-up and refuel from workouts
- lose weight, if desired, and maintain energy for running
- feel better, run better, and thereby feel better about yourself

This balance sheet approach can be particularly helpful to marathoners who feel tired all the time. It can help you understand *why* you are tired. For example:

- If you skip meals and deposit nothing into your daily calorie account at breakfast and lunch, you can clearly see why you lack energy for your afternoon training session.
- If you are a weight-conscious runner or walker, calorie information allows you to determine how much food you should eat for fuel yet still lose body fat.
- If you are a food-lover who exercises to be able to eat more, the calorie guidelines indicate how much you can eat guilt-free!

Hungry marathoners need good food on a regular schedule. Why skimp on daytime meals and feel tired all day, only to spend your whole calorie budget in the evening? This calorie-budgeting system encourages you to eat and to eat enough at breakfast and lunch to support both an active life and a rigorous

How many calories do marathoners require? By using the following formula, you can estimate your personal calorie needs and gain a perspective on how to balance calories eaten versus calories expended.*

1. *To determine your resting metabolic rate, that is, the amount of calories you need to simply breathe, pump blood, and be alive:*

   Multiply your weight by 10 calories per pound (or 22 calories per kilogram).

   For example, if you weigh 120 pounds, you need approximately 1,200 calories (120 x 10) to simply do nothing all day except exist. If you are significantly overweight, use an adjusted weight: the weight that is half-way between your desired weight and your current weight.

2. *Add more calories for general daily activity apart from your running and other purposeful exercise:*

   If you are moderately active throughout the day, add about 50 percent of your resting metabolic rate.

   If you are sedentary, add a little less than 50 percent; if very active, a little more.

   For example, a moderately active 120-pound woman who requires 1,200 calories for her resting metabolic rate needs about another 600 calories for activities of daily living. This totals 1,800 calories per day—without running.

3. *Add more calories for your purposeful exercise:*

   The general rule of thumb is 100 calories per mile, but more precisely, this depends upon your weight. If you weight more than 130 pounds, add a few more calories. If you weight less, subtract a few, or go by these approximate guidelines:

Weight, lbs (kg)	Calories per mile
120 (55)	95
140 (64)	110
160 (73)	125
180 (82)	140

   Hence, if you are a 120-pound woman who runs five miles per day, you burn about 475 calories while running. This brings you to about 2,275 calories per day to maintain your weight. For simplicity, let's just say 2,300 calories.

4. *If you want to lose weight, subtract 20 percent of your total calorie needs:*

   .20 x 2,300 calories = 460 calories

   2,300 - 460 calories = 1,840 calories, or more simply 1,800 calories total per day

(Refer to Chapter 14 for more guidance on weight loss.)

5. *Now, take your calorie budget and divide it into three parts of the day:*

For the 120-pound woman on a diet, this comes to 600 calories per section of the day:

Breakfast/snack	600
Lunch/snack	600
Dinner/snack	600

Or, for four meals per day:

Breakfast	500
Lunch	500
Lunch #2	300
Dinner	500

6. *The next step is to read food labels to become familiar with the calorie content of the foods you commonly eat and then fuel your body according to the rules for a well-balanced diet.*

Here are approximate calorie needs for marathoners of different weights who are moderately active throughout the day:

Weight lbs (kg)	Calorie needs for: daily living	with 5-mile run or walk	with 10-mile run or walk
120 (55)	1,800	2,300	2,700
140 (64)	2,100	2,650	3,200
160 (73)	2,400	3,000	3,650
180 (82)	2,700	3,400	4,100

*These guidelines do not address the needs of each individual. For personalized calorie information you should meet with a registered dietitian who specializes in sports nutrition. Contact the American Dietetic Association at (800) 366-1655 to find a sports nutritionist in your area, or visit their website at www.eatright.org and use the convenient referral network.

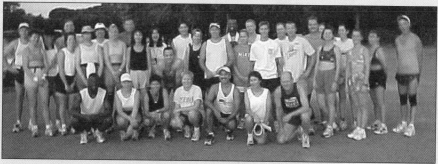

Marathoners come in all sizes and shapes and have different calorie requirements. By knowing your personal calorie budget, you can fuel your muscles optimally to maintain high energy.

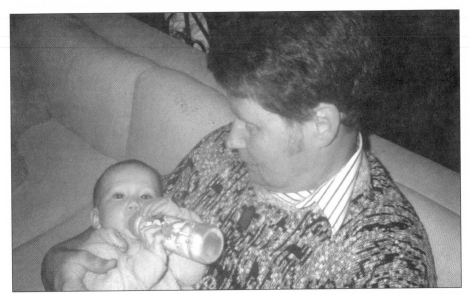

Infants have the natural ability to eat when they are hungry and stop when they are content. Many adults, however, have lost this ability. Calorie knowledge can help adults relearn how to eat appropriately.

training program. Without a doubt, if you consume calories evenly throughout the day by eating a variety of wholesome foods, you will invest in high energy, added stamina, strength, and smooth running, to say nothing of better health.

Many marathoners can naturally regulate a proper calorie intake and have little need to calculate calories. They simply eat when they are hungry and stop when they are content. Others have lost touch with their body's ability to regulate an appropriate food intake; they starve, then stuff themselves. They often do not eat when they are hungry (such as happens with severe reducing diets), but then overeat later on. Counting calories is particularly helpful for these marathoners who have trouble regulating their food intake. They can use calories as a crutch to help them 1) get in touch with appropriate portion sizes and 2) acknowledge how they feel when they are appropriately fed. Once educated, they can then naturally regulate their food intake—without counting calories.

● **HONOR HUNGER**—The more you exercise, the hungrier you will get. Whereas most marathoners simply honor their hunger and refuel with wholesome meals, other marathoners feel confused

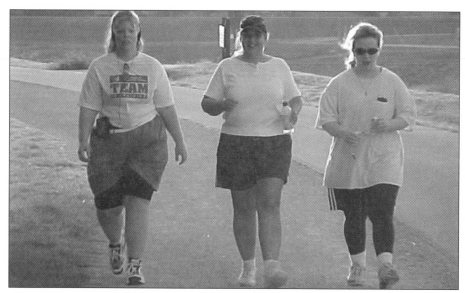

Large marathoners require more calories than do their lighter peers. If you have substantial body weight to carry, fuel yourself adequately so you can better enjoy your exercise program.

by hunger and sometimes even feel guilty that they are always eager to eat. One walker perceived her hunger as being bad and wrong. Hunger is normal; it is simply your body's way of talking to you, requesting fuel. Plan to eat at least every four hours.

You should not spend your day feeling hungry—even if you are on a reducing diet (see Chapter 14) If your 8:00 A.M. breakfast finds you hungry earlier than noon, your breakfast simply contained too few calories. You need a supplemental midmorning snack or a bigger breakfast that supplies about one-third of your day's calories.

Come noontime, instead of feeling that something is wrong with you because you are hungry again, enjoy lunch as being the second-most-important meal of the day. Morning runners, in particular, need a hearty lunch to refuel their muscles; afternoon runners need a respectable lunch and afternoon snack to fuel-up for their after-work training. Ideally, lunch and snacks should provide about one-third of your day's calories.

Whereas some runners like to satisfy their appetites with big meals, others prefer to divide their calories into mini-meals eaten every two hours. That's fine, if that's your preference and better suits your training schedule and lifestyle.

CHAPTER 14

Weight and Marathoners

EXERCISE BURNS CALORIES! AND THAT'S WHY MANY PEOPLE WALK, run, and enjoy other forms of activity. Consistent exercise helps them manage their weight and allows more freedom with eating. For some walkers and runners, however, weight remains a significant issue. As coach Lloyd Burnett of Mission, TX said, "I once trained three new marathoners who each lost 20 pounds in less than 6 months. Each of them made the commitment to be conscious about their calories and overall food intake. My training partner and I, on the other hand, have run almost 20 marathons but we each still weigh 220 pounds. I love my beer and he loves his tortillas. We're not willing to commit to the diet part of the event, even though we see the results all around us."

● **HOW TO LOSE WEIGHT AND HAVE ENERGY TO EXERCISE**—I spend hours helping marathoners who struggle to lose weight. Most feel frustrated that they just can't seem to shed those final few pounds. Inevitably, the first words they say to me are, "I know what I *should* do to lose weight. I just can't do it." They think they should follow a strict diet with rigid rules and regulations.

Wrong. Diets don't work. If diets did work, every marathoner would be as thin as desired.

> **❝ I suggest that people spend a year trying all the different diets they can find. Then, after having no success at achieving their goals, they gradually modify their normal eating habits. There are no quick fixes for weight loss. Period. Show me a quick fix, and I will show you how you are hurting your body. ❞**
>
> John Correia, San Diego, CA
> Coach, Team in Training

Although only nature knows the best weight for your body, the following guidelines offer a very general method to estimate a healthy weight. For a weight range, add or subtract 10 percent, according to your body frame and musculature.

Women: 100 pounds for the first 5 feet of height;
    5 pounds per inch thereafter

Men: 106 pounds for the first 5 feet of height;
    6 pounds per inch thereafter

Although marathoners commonly want to be lighter than the average person, heed this message: If you are striving to weigh significantly less than the weight estimated by this general guideline, think again. Pay attention to the genetic design for your body and don't struggle to get too light. The best weight goal is to be *fit* and *healthy* rather than sleek and skinny. Even fat marathoners can be fit and healthy!

The key to losing weight is to:
- stop thinking about *going* on a diet and
- start learning *how to eat healthfully.*

Marsha, a novice marathoner, thought skimping on food was a good way to diet and she felt frustrated by her lack of weight loss. She explained, "I don't eat breakfast. I run at lunchtime and then just eat a yogurt and a banana. Nighttime is my trouble-time. I eat everything in sight. Cookies are my downfall. It seems the more I diet, the more weight I gain."

Clearly, *not eating* was Marsha's problem. Dieting and denial were getting her nowhere. I reminded Marsha that she is *supposed* to eat and encouraged her to trust that appropriate eating will contribute to an appropriate weight.

> ❝ *I have been walking marathons for two years. Like the majority of walkers, I was hoping to lose weight, but that has not been the case for me. Many of my walking friends have even gained weight. Exercise alone does not suffice!* ❞
>
> Becky Goodrum, Cleveland, OH

● **HOW MUCH IS OK TO EAT?**—As I outlined in Chapter 13, active people need more than a few calories to fuel themselves. To determine just how much you can appropriately eat, refer back to page 102. Note that your body requires an amazing amount of energy to pump blood, breathe, produce urine, grow hair, and simply exist. Also note that you deserve to eat those maintenance calories even if you are injured and unable to run.

An appropriate reducing diet knocks off *only 20 percent of your calorie needs.* Many weight-conscious marathoners try to eat as little as possible. That's a big mistake. Perhaps the following case study will help you understand why.

Ann, a 120-pound nurse, walks 5 miles most days. She requires about 2,200 to 2,300 calories to maintain her weight:
- 1,200 calories for her resting metabolic rate
  (10 calories per pound x 120 pounds)
- 600 calories for general daily activity (50% x 1,200 calories)
- 475 calories for her walk (95 calories per mile x 5 miles)

To appropriately lose weight, I recommended she cut her total calorie intake by 20 percent (about 400 to 500 calories), leaving her with 1,800 calories for her reducing diet.

> *I frequently see people gain weight during marathon training. They believe the training gives them license to eat anything and everything. Unfortunately, a 3,000-calorie dessert still shows up on the butt.*
>
> John Correia, San Diego CA
> Coach, Team in Training

To Ann, 1,800 sounded like too many calories. She exclaimed "I could never eat that much without turning into a blimp. If I can't lose weight when I'm on a 1,000-calorie diet, how could I possibly do so on 1,800? My metabolism is *so slow.* I seem to gain weight just smelling cookies."

Although Ann challenged my calorie recommendations, I suggested that she keep an open mind. The latest research on athletes' calorie needs suggest that very few athletes actually do have slow metabolisms. Researchers have even studied active people like Ann who claim to maintain weight despite eating next to nothing. When carefully monitored, these women burned the calories one would expect based on standard calculations. Their metabolisms were fine, but they had problems acknowledging how much food they actually ate. Their nibbles on bagels, apples, rice cakes, and broken cookie added up! (For more information, refer to *Slow Metabolism Woes* in Chapter 16.)

Because Ann claimed she ate far less than her peers, I suggested she heighten her awareness of her food intake by keeping food records. Food records can be extremely useful to help you understand your eating habits. For example, by listing *everything* that you eat, you might notice that you:

- eat when reading and don't even notice the portion
- eat too little at breakfast and lunch, only to overeat at night
- diet Monday through Thursday, then splurge on weekends.

Accurate food records can help you lose weight because you'll likely end up eating about 20 percent less, which, after all, is an appropriate reducing diet!

● **FIVE KEYS TO SUCCESSFUL WEIGHT REDUCTION**—Using your calorie guidelines, you can lose weight with the following five keys to successful weight reduction.

Key #1. Eat enough. Don't get too hungry or you'll blow your diet. For example, Lori, a receptionist and a runner, tried to self-impose the following bare-bones diet:

Breakfast:	coffee	0 calories
Lunch:	dry salad	100
Snack:	large apple	150
Dinner:	frozen diet meal	300
Total calories:		*550*

This totaled *less than a quarter* of the 2,400 calories she required. No wonder she lacked energy for running. She'd often skip workouts and then at night eat everything in sight, only to get up the next morning with a food hangover. She'd then vow to get back on her diet, skip breakfast, skimp on lunch, lack energy to enjoy running, and blow her diet again at night. Although Lori deserved a lot of credit for having the willpower to survive the day on 550 calories, her method was mistaken. Her diet was too strict.

If you, like Lori, are trying to lose weight by eating as little as possible and exercising as hard as you can, remember that the less you eat, the more likely you are to blow your diet. Even if you can successfully restrict your intake, the less you eat, the more your body adjusts to having fewer calories. You will start to hibernate similar to what a bear does in winter when food is scarce. That is, your metabolic rate will drop to conserve calories and you'll feel lethargic, cold, and lack energy to exercise.

Research comparing dieters who either crash-dieted or followed a more reasonable reducing plan showed that both groups lost the same amount of body fat. The strict diet, however, caused the metabolic rate to drop. Why bother to eat next to nothing when you can lose weight with eating just 20 percent less than you need to maintain your weight?

Most of my clients follow 1,800- to 2,200-calorie reduction diets. This is far more than most 800- to 1,200-calorie diets that are designed for sedentary people who can get away with eating very little. You need a substantial amount of energy to fuel your muscles and have energy to enjoy your training.

Key #2. Be sure that you eat more during the day, so that you'll be able to eat less (diet) at night. For an appropriate reducing program, I recommend that you divide your calories evenly throughout the day. Because athletes tend to get hungry at least every four hours, an appropriate reduction diet for a 120-pound female marathoner might be:

Breakfast:	8 A.M.	500 calories
Lunch:	Noon	500
Snack:	4 P.M.	300
Run:	6 P.M.	
Dinner:	8 P.M.	500

Your goal is to eat on a schedule to *prevent* yourself from getting too hungry. I call this my "eat more, lose weight" food plan.

Your training program may require creative meal scheduling if you exercise during meal times. For example, if you exercise at 6 P.M.—potentially at the height of your hunger—you might better enjoy your training if you eat part of your dinner beforehand. For example, trade in your 200-calorie dinner potato for a 200-calorie bagel at 4 P.M. Similarly, if you exercise at 6:00 A.M., you might enjoy greater energy if you eat part of your breakfast beforehand, such as a slice of toast and a glass of juice, and then eat the rest afterwards to recover from the workout and satisfy your hunger. (As I mentioned in Chapter 8, you need to experiment with pre-exercise food to determine the right amount of calories that boost your energy without making you feel heavy and sluggish.)

Some marathoners believe that exercising "on empty"—for example, running first thing in the morning before breakfast— helps them to burn more body fat. While this is true, keep in mind that *burning* body fat does not equate to *losing* body fat. To have a *net loss* of body fat, you need to create a calorie *deficit*; that is, you need to burn more calories than you consume over a period of days. People who exercise on empty have difficulty creating and maintaining a calorie deficit because:

- they lack the energy for long, strong workouts, and end up burning fewer calories than someone who is properly fueled before exercise and
- they experience extreme hunger later on, which can lead to overeating calories.

Key #3. Eat an appropriate amount of fat. If you are currently eating a high-fat diet filled with butter, mayonnaise, salad dressing, greasy meals, and rich desserts, you should cut back on these fattening foods. Excess dietary fat easily turns into excess body fat, if not clogged arteries.

But many of today's runners avoid fat. They think that if they eat fat, they'll instantly get fat. Not always the case. Take

● STOP BLOWING YOUR DIET!

If blown diets are your downfall, I recommend you take the following steps:

- Experiment with eating bigger breakfasts and lunches.

- Plan a substantial afternoon snack or second lunch, especially if you won't be eating dinner until after 7 P.M.

- "Diet" at night by eating smaller portions than usual.

Question: "I walk four miles every day and eat only foods with no fat in them. I haven't lost any weight. What am I doing wrong?"

Answer: Pam was eating 2,400 calories of fat-free foods, oblivious to their calories. She required only 2,200 calories per day.

Pam's overall diet was very limited, unbalanced, and boring. Every day, she ate the following items:

Breakfast	2 apples
Lunch	1 bagel, 1 apple
Snack	1 apple, 10 dutch pretzels
Dinner	2 bagels, 2 apples

Total intake: 2,400 calories of fat-free snacks

Daily needs: 2,200 calories

I suggested that Pam subtract half of the apples, bagels, and pretzels and replace those calories with peanut butter, cheese, and tuna with low-fat mayonnaise. This way she could:
- boost her protein intake for a more balanced diet
- satisfy her appetite
- reduce her desire to eat yet another bagel (with yet more calories) and reduce her overall calorie intake
- She did, and this helped her successfully meet her weight goals.

a look around and notice the number of trim marathoners whose diets include some fat.

If you are trying to knock *all* the fat out of your diet, think again and see Chapter 6. Some fat in your food may actually help you *lose* weight. Runners who try to eat a no-fat diet:
- commonly feel hungry, denied, deprived
- feel guilty when they inevitably "cheat" by eating fat
- eat an unbalanced diet that may be too low in protein and can hurt their performance.

One study showed that dieters who were instructed to eat 1,200 calories of a high-fat diet actually lost more body fat than the group who were instructed to eat 1,200 calories of a very-low-fat diet. Why? Because the high-fat dieters were better able to comply with their regimen. Fat can be helpful for dieters because it takes longer to digest and provides a nice feeling of satisfaction that can prevent you from searching through the kitchen, scrounging for something tasty to eat.

You'll enjoy better luck with reducing body fat if you give yourself a reasonable calorie and fat budget to spend on the foods that you want to eat. By choosing the 25-percent-fat diet that I described in Chapter 6, you can add a little fat to each meal, feel less hungry, and be better able to stick to your diet. For generations, people have lost fat even though their diets included fat. You can too!

Key #4. Don't try to lose weight every day. Maintaining can be O.K. Losing weight requires enough mental energy to tell yourself, "I'd rather be thinner than eat more calories." Some days you may lack that mental energy. For example, Paul, a lawyer and runner who wanted to lose five pounds before the Chicago Marathon, was stressed out by his demanding work load, training schedule, and family problems. Although he wanted to drop a few pounds, he lacked the mental energy he needed to cut calories. At the end of the day, he'd inevitably succumb to ice cream. It seemed like a nice reward for having survived the day, but it also contributed to weight gain.

● WHY ARE YOU EATING?

Food has many roles. It satisfies hunger, fuels muscles, is a pleasurable part of social gatherings and celebrations, rewards us at the end of a stressful day, and has a calming effect. If you tend to eat for reasons other than fuel, think HALT and ask yourself, Why do I want to eat? Is it because I am:
- **H**ungry?
- **A**ngry or Anxious?
- **L**onely?
- **T**ired?

If you are eating inappropriately, remember that no amount of food will solve any problem. Don't start eating if you know you'll have problems stopping.

I reminded Paul that he is only human, with a limited amount of mental and physical energy. Rather than punish himself for lacking energy to diet, he needed to accept the fact that he was stressed and in need of comfort. Like it or not, food provided that comfort.

I recommended that Paul let go of his current goal to *lose* fat and focus instead on *maintaining* his weight and fueling his muscles appropriately. Well-fueled muscles would enhance his running more than would poorly fueled muscles, especially if they were depleted from improper dieting. I also reminded Paul he has the rest of his life to lose excess body fat. In this already stressful season in his life, he might be happier removing the additional self-imposed stress of trying to lose weight. He reluctantly agreed with that reality.

Stressful times are often poor times to try to reduce body fat. Rather, focus on exercising regularly to help cope with stress and on eating healthfully to prevent the weight gain that sometimes occurs during stressful times. Eat every four hours to keep your appetite under control. Note that marathoners who are both stressed and hungry can easily succumb to overeating. But no amount of food will solve any problem. In fact, it only adds to your feeling out of control.

> **" Do not be obsessed with the numbers on the scale. With time and training, you will learn at what weight you can perform well. Listening to your body is more accurate than any scale. "**
>
> Mike Czech, Edison, NJ
> Coach, Team in Training

Key #6. Have realistic weight goals. Weight is more than a matter of willpower; genetics plays a large role. If you are eating appropriately during the day, exercising regularly, eating lighter at night, and waking up eager for breakfast but still have not lost weight, perhaps you have an unrealistic goal. It's possible that you have no excess fat to lose and are already very lean for your genetic blueprint. Like it or not, weight is somewhat controlled by genetics. Although you might wish for a sleeker physique, nature may want you to look more like a discus thrower!

Marsha, the novice marathoner, was short and had thin hair and big thighs, "just like my mothers and sisters." Although she put no effort into trying to grow taller or thicken her hair, she obsessed about the fat on her thighs and spent

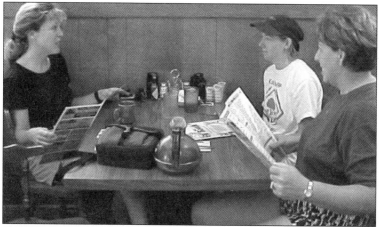

Eating in restaurants need not be a dietary downfall. The trick is: don't "save calories" so you get too hungry and then order foods that fail to help you meet your weight goals. If you enter a restaurant feeling only slightly hungry; you'll be able to order foods wisely!

lots of energy trying to reduce them.

I reminded Marsha that although she could remodel her body to a certain extent, she couldn't totally redesign it. Plain and simple, walkers and runners, like fruits, come in varying sizes and shapes. No one body type is right or wrong.

In order to determine an appropriate weight for your body, I recommend you stop looking at the scale and start looking at your family. Imagine yourself at a family reunion:

- How do you compare to other members of your family?
- Are you currently leaner than they are? fatter? the same?
- If leaner, are you straining to stay that way?
- If you are significantly leaner, you may already be underfat for your body.

I counsel many runners who put their lives on hold, struggling to lose a final few pounds. As Marsha said as she grabbed onto her thighs, "I hate being seen in running shorts. But no matter how much I exercise, I can't get rid of these fat thighs. I must be doing something wrong."

Marsha was simply trying to get to a weight that was abnormal for her genetics. She was already leaner that other members of her family. I helped her to understand the reason why women (as compared to men) have "fat thighs": the fat in the thigh area is sex-specific. It is a storehouse of energy for potential pregnancy and breast feeding and is *supposed* to be there. Just as women have breast tissue, women also have thigh tissue. Women have fatter thighs than men because women are *women*. Marsha needed to accept the realities of being a woman and stop comparing herself to the magazine models who indeed have rare physiques.

If you are wasting time complaining about your body, keep in perspective:

• Life is a gift.

• Life is too short to be spent obsessing about food and weight. Yes, you do want to be fit and healthy, but you need not strive to be sleek and skinny. The cost attached to achieving the perfect weight and the perfect body is often yo-yo dieting, poor nutrition, lack of energy to exercise, guilt for eating, a sense of failure that can play havoc with your self-esteem, and, of course, poor marathon performance.

Planned weight loss—one to two pounds per week—and marathon training don't mix. The weight loss should occur prior to or during the early stages of the train-ing program. Once mileage and quality of training increase, the nutrition focus should be on replenishment, not deficit, of calories.

Ronnie Carda, Madison, WI
Coach, Team in Training

• **SUMMARY**—Food is fuel, healthful, and health-giving. You are supposed to eat even if you are trying to lose weight. Be realistic about your expectations and remember:

• The thinnest marathoner may not be the fastest marathoner.

• The best fueled marathoners will always win with good nutrition.

Also remember the following keys to successful weight control:

• You are supposed to eat even if you want to lose body fat. Deduct only 20 percent of your calorie budget, but don't starve yourself.

• You need to eat during the day, then diet at night. Morning hunger is a sign you didn't overeat the night before.

• Your diet can appropriately include a little bit of fat to keep you from feeling hungry and also from feeling denied.

• You don't have to *lose* weight every day; stress-filled days can be for *maintaining* weight.

• Be realistic with your weight goals. You may have no weight to lose, according to your genetics.

CHAPTER 15

How to Gain Weight Healthfully

F YOU ARE AMONG THE MINORITY OF MARATHONERS WHO STRUGGLE with being too thin, food may seem a medicine, meals a burden, and the expense of food budget-breaking. Through discipline and diet, you can change your physique to a certain extent, but first, have a clear picture of your genetic blueprint and a realistic goal:

- What do other people in your family look like?
- Was your mother or father very slim at your age?
- When did s/he gain weight?
- What does s/he look like now?

If at your age, a parent was equally thin, you probably are genetically predisposed to be thin and may have trouble adding pounds. Some people are simply "hard gainers." For example, in an overfeeding study on identical twins, some pairs of twins gained more weight than others, despite the fact that everyone overate by an equal amount—1,000 extra calories per day. In another study, some subjects who theoretically should have gained eleven pounds during a month-long overfeeding study gained an average of only six pounds. Why the difference? No one knows. One guess is some people fidget more than others and this fidgeting can burn an extra 300 to 700 calories per day.

● **SIX RULES FOR GAINING WEIGHT**—If you are a hard gainer, you may require a significant amount of calories to add weight. There is no instant cure or magic solution. The bottom line is you have to consume more calories than you expend. Adding muscle-building exercise such as weightlifting helps convert the extra calories into muscle rather than fat.

I encourage underweight marathoners to consume an additional 500 to 1,000 calories per day. If you are committed to the weight-gain process, you can expect to gain one-half to one pound per week, perhaps more depending on your age. For example, high school and collegiate athletes may bulk-up more easily than the fully mature 35-year-old who is genetically skinny.

The trick to successful weight gain is to pay careful attention to these six important rules.

1. *Eat consistently.* Have three hearty meals plus one or two additional snacks daily. Do *not* skip meals! You may not feel hungry for lunch if you've had a big breakfast, but you should eat regardless. Otherwise, you'll miss out on important calories that you need to accomplish your goal.

2. *Eat larger portions.* Some people think they need to buy expensive weight-gain powders. They don't need special powders; standard food works fine. The only reason commercial powders "work" is because they provide additional calories. For example, one marathoner religiously drank the recommended three glasses per day of a 300-calorie weight-gain shake. This gave him an extra 900 calories and the desired results. Although he credited the weight-gain formula for his success, he could have less expensively consumed those calories with supermarket foods. I suggested that he invest his food budget in readily available foods:

- a bigger bowl of cereal
- a larger piece of fruit
- an extra sandwich for lunch or a large sub sandwich
- three potatoes at dinner instead of two
- a taller glass of milk.

When he did this, he met his goal of 1,000 extra calories per day and continued to see the desired results.

3. *Select higher calorie foods, but not higher fat foods.* Excess fat calories easily convert into body fat that fattens you up rather than bulks up your muscles. They also diminish your appetite. The best bet for extra calories is to choose carbohydrate-rich foods that have more calories than an equally enjoyable counterpart (see sidebar, *How to Boost Your Calories*). These extra carbohydrates will give you the energy you need to do muscle-building exercise. By reading food labels, you'll be able to make the best choices.

4. *Drink lots of juice and low-fat milk.* Beverages are a simple way to increase your calorie intake. Instead of drinking primarily water, quench your thirst with calorie-containing fluids. One high school athlete gained 13 pounds over the summer by simply adding six glasses of cranapple juice (about 1,000 calories) to his standard daily diet. Extra juices are not only a great source of calories and fluids but also of carbohydrates to keep your muscles well fueled.

5. *Do strength training* (push-ups, weightlifting) to stimulate muscular development, so that you bulk up instead of fatten up. Note that extra *exercise,* not extra protein, is the key to muscular development. If you are concerned the extra exercise will result in weight loss rather than weight gain, remember that exercise tends to stimulate the appetite. Yes, a hard run

● HOW TO BOOST YOUR CALORIES

Choose more:	Calories	Instead of:	Calories
Cranberry juice, 8 ounces	170	Orange juice, 8 ounces	110
Grape juice, 8 ounces	160	Grapefruit juice, 8 ounces	100
Banana, 1 large	170	Apple, 1 large	130
Granola, 1½ cups	780	Bran flakes, 1½ cups	200
Grape-Nuts, 1½ cups	660	Cheerios, 1½ cups	160
Corn, 1 cup	140	Green beans, 1 cup	40
Carrots, 1 cup	45	Zucchini, 1 cup	30
Split pea soup, 1 cup	130	Vegetable soup, 1 cup	80
Baked beans, 1 cup	260	Rice, 1 cup	190

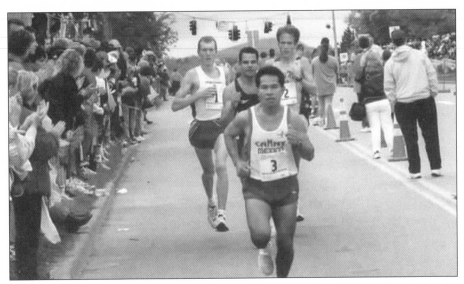

Even among the top finishers, runners come in different sizes and shapes. Some are short and stocky; others are lean and lanky.

may temporarily "kill" your appetite right after the workout because your body temperature is elevated, but within a few hours when you have cooled down, you will be plenty hungry. The more you exercise, the more you'll want to eat—*assuming you make the time to do so.*

6. Be patient. If you are in high school or college and don't easily bulk up this year, you may do so more easily as you get older. Know that you can be a strong marathoner by being well fueled and well trained. Your skinny legs may hurt your self-esteem more than your athletic ability.

CHAPTER 16

Women and Weight

ACTIVE WOMEN OF ALL AGES AND ABILITIES APPRECIATE THE FIT-
ness, fun, and physical benefits that come with walking,
running, and other forms of training for the marathon. To support their exercise programs, women clearly benefit from good
nutrition to help them:

- attain their goal of completing a marathon
- maintain energy to handle their fast-paced lifestyles
- ensure having regular menstrual periods
- reduce the risk of injuries.

Due to the prevailing myths that thinness contributes to
both better performance and happiness, some female and male
marathoners consider food to be a fattening enemy rather than
a friendly fuel. With the fear that eating meals will make them
heavy and slow, they deny themselves permission to eat adequately. Appropriate meals are placed on hold until those final
few pounds get lost and the dieter begins to feel better about
her weight.

Fueled by the "thinner is better" philosophy, the female
marathoners who strive to be abnormally thin commonly pay a
high price: poor nutrition, poorly fueled muscles, loss of menses,
stress fractures and other injuries, to say nothing of reduced stamina, endurance, and performance. In their overconcern about
their weight, they forget this formula for success:

appropriate eating + regular exercise = appropriate weight

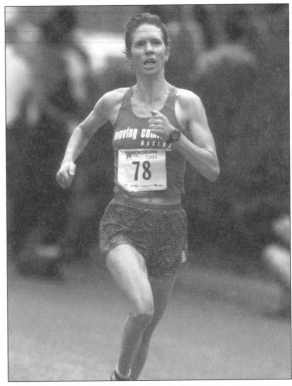

Women can be lean, fit and healthy. Earlier in her running career, Bakoulis thought being lighter would help her be a better runner. She now knows being stronger and well fueled is more important.

Whereas Chapter 14 offered guidance about how to lose weight and maintain energy for walking or running, this chapter provides an additional perspective to help resolve the special food and weight concerns of active women. If you are a man who struggles with food, the information can help you, as well.

Clearly, weight is a bigger issue for women than for men. Let's look the possible explanations.

1. Women are supposed to have more body fat than men. Plain and simple, nature prescribes to women a certain amount of body fat that is essential for two reasons:
• to protect their ability to create and nourish healthy babies
• to be a storehouse of calories for pregnancy and breast feeding

This essential body fat is stored not only in the breasts but also in the hips, abdomen, and upper legs. That's why women tend to have heavier thighs than most men.

Whereas 11 to 13 percent of a woman's body weight is essential fat stores, only 3 to 5 percent of a man's body weight is essential body fat. Hence, women who try to achieve the "cut look" of male athletes create physiological turmoil and often have to pay the price by starving, bingeing, and obsessing about food in order to reach their desired image.

2. Women commonly target an unnatural weight. Women who try to get below their natural weight are the ones most likely to struggle with food and fight the battle with the bulge. Given that even some of those very lean, front-of-the-pack women runners wish they could be lighter, I'm not surprised that eating disorders abound. The majority of male runners, in comparison, seem to be more at peace with their natural weight and, consequently, at peace with food.

3. Women hold distorted body images. The Madison Avenue image that adorns every storefront and magazine ad leads us to believe that nature makes all women universally lean. Any aberration is thought to be a result of gluttony and lack of willpower. Wrong!

Nature makes us in different sizes and shapes, like it or not. If the marathoners who are discontent with their weight could only learn to accept and love their bodies, eating disorders would be rare. As one food-obsessed woman—5'7" and 115 pounds—lamented, "I don't have the gaunt look of the really fast runners. I really wish I could weigh 110." She was unable to see that she was already very lean. A normal, healthy weight for a 5'7" woman is 135 pounds! She was training harder and harder to burn calories and lose body fat. Her running contrasted with that of other runners, commonly men, who train primarily to enhance performance, not to reshape their bodies.

> ❝ *As a runner who has gained weight as I've gotten older, I've had to come to peace with my heavier body. I feel less perfect, less in control. I'm learning to love my body from the inside out and be thankful for all the wonderful things it does for me, like finish marathons.* ❞
>
> Cynthia Harding, Boston, MA

● THE SLOW METABOLISM WOES—Some women comment that the fitter they are, the fewer calories they need. As marathoner Priscilla Welch once said, "I'm amazed at what nonrunners can tuck away." These comments raise questions about metabolic efficiency. Does nature slow a female athlete's metabolism to protect her from getting too thin and having inadequate fat stores to support pregnancy?

Frustration with inability to lose weight abounds among women who claim they have a slow metabolism and eat less than they "deserve," given their rigorous daily exercise regimen. Perhaps you've heard your buddies express complaints similar to the following:

• I eat less than my friends but I still don't lose weight. There must be something wrong with my metabolism.
• I maintain weight on only 1,000 calories per day. I want to lose a few pounds, but I can't imagine eating any less.
• I run at least eight miles every day and eat only one meal a day. I can't understand why I don't lose weight.

What's going on? Is it true that some marathoners are "energy-efficient"? Do they efficiently utilize every calorie that enters their body so they are able to maintain weight on fewer calories than their counterparts who more unproductively burn them off? According to Dr. Jack Wilmore, exercise physiologist at the University of Texas at Austin, the energy-efficient athlete does not exist. His research suggests that metabolic rate is closely tied to muscle mass. Because many women who restrict calories end up burning muscle tissue for energy, they tend to have less muscle mass. Consequently, they require fewer calories. "Plain and simple, athletes who have well-developed muscles require more calories than those who have less muscle."

Other researchers challenge the energy-efficiency theory, believing that a slower metabolism may be nature's way to conserve calories. After all, the women who perceive themselves as being energy-efficient commonly complain about being cold all the time, feeling lethargic, and lacking regular menstrual cycles. These symptoms suggest that their diet is too meager to support normal body functions.

While the debate continues, your solution comes in finding

the right amount of calories and nutrients to support a healthy weight for your body.

● **WOMEN, RUNNING, AND AMENORRHEA**—If you are a marathoner who previously had regular menstrual periods but currently has stopped menstruating, you are experiencing *amenorrhea*. Although you may think the loss of menses is because you are too thin or are exercising too much, thinness and exercise may not be the causes of amenorrhea. After all, many very thin marathoners *do* have regular menses.

Studies have shown that both regularly menstruating and amenorrheic athletes commonly have the same amount of body fat. Clearly, leanness and intense exercise are not the simple explanation to the complexities of amenorrhea. But the question remains unanswered: Why, given a group of women who have a similar training program and the same low percent of body fat, do some experience menstrual problems and others don't?

Marathoners with amenorrhea often strive to maintain an unhealthy low weight. If you perceive yourself as struggling harder than your counterparts to maintain your desired leanness, note that the cost of achieving that leanness is likely inadequate nutrition and, consequently, loss of menses. Athletic amenorrhea is commonly a nutritional problem and sometimes a red flag for an eating disorder. If you stop having regular menstrual periods, be sure to consult with both your gynecologist and sports nutritionist for professional guidance.

● RISK FACTORS FOR AMENORRHEA

You are more likely to stop having regular menstrual periods if you have any of the following:
- a restrictive diet
- a rapid weight loss
- low body weight
- low percent body fat
- a rigorous exercise program
- irregular menstrual periods even before you started to train hard
- significant emotional stress

About 24 to 26 percent of competitive runners experience amenorrhea. Runners aren't the only women with menstrual problems. Others include:
- 19 to 44 percent of ballet dancers
- 12 percent of both collegiate swimmers and world-class cyclists
- 3 to 5 percent of the general female population

● **HEALTH RISKS**—Although you may deem amenorrhea a desirable side effect of exercise because you no longer have to deal with the hassles and possible discomfort of monthly menstrual periods, amenorrhea can lead to undesirable problems that can interfere with your health and ability to perform at your best. These problems include:
- almost a three times higher incidence of stress fractures
- premature osteoporosis (weakening of the bones) that can effect your bone health in the not-too-distant future
- possible higher risk of heart disease
- inability to conceive should you want to have a baby.

If the amenorrhea is caused by anorexia, it is a symptom of pain and unhappiness in your life. Note that the "absence of at least three consecutive menstrual cycles" is part of the American Psychiatric Association's definition for anorexia.

Amenorrheic women who resume menses do restore some of the bone density lost during their months of amenorrhea, particularly if they are younger than seventeen years. But they do not restore all of it. Your goal should be to minimize the damages of amenorrhea by eating appropriately and taking the proper steps to regain your menstrual periods. Remember: Food is fuel, healthful and health-giving, not a fattening enemy.

● **RESOLVING AMENORRHEA**—The possible changes required to resume menses include:
- training 5 to 15 percent less (50 minutes instead of an hour)
- consuming 10 percent more calories each week, until you ingest an appropriate amount given your activity level. For example, if you have been eating 1,500 calories a day, eat 150 more calories

per day for a total of 1,650 total calories a day during the first week; eat a total of 1800 calories per day the second week; 1,950 the third week, and so on. (See Chapter 13 for how to determine an appropriate calorie intake.)

- choosing more protein-rich foods, particularly red meat
- gaining a few pounds

Some amenorrheic runners have resumed menses with just reduced exercise and no weight gain. Those who totally stop training, such as happens at the time of an injury, often resume menses within two months. Others resume menstruating after gaining less than five pounds. And despite what you may think, this small amount of weight gain does not result in your "getting fat" and can be enough to achieve better health.

If you have stopped menstruating and believe that poor eating may be part of the problem, you should consider getting a nutrition checkup with a registered dietitian who specializes in sports nutrition (see the sidebar on page 128, *Steps to Resolve Eating Disorders*).

The following tips may help you resume menses or at least rule out nutrition-related factors.

1. *Throw away the bathroom scale.* Rather than striving to achieve a certain number on the scale, let your body weigh what it weighs. Focus on how healthy you feel and how well you perform, rather than on the number you weigh. Remember: Weight is influenced by genetics and is more than just a matter of willpower or a "numbers game."

2. *If you have weight to lose, don't crash-diet but rather moderately cut back on your food intake by about 20 percent.* Severe dieters commonly lose their menstrual periods, suggesting that

> **I loved being very light, lean, and free of menstrual cramps. That is, until I got a stress fracture, then another and another. My poor diet had caught up with me.**
>
> **I saw a dietitian who helped me normalize my eating. I started to have more yogurt, cottage cheese and tuna. I even added some peanut butter. Instead of "getting fat" (my biggest fear), I actually started to feel stronger and run better. When I got my period three months later, I was relieved to know my body was healthier inside and functioning the way it should.**
>
> Cynthia Harding, Boston, MA

If you think that you are struggling too much with food and have an eating disorder, seek help and information by contacting:

National Eating Disorders Association
603 Stewart St., Suite 803
Seattle, WA 98101
Tel: (206) 382-3587
www.NationalEatingDisorders.org

American Dietetic Association
216 W. Jackson Blvd. #800
Chicago, IL 60606-6995
Tel: (800)-877-1600
www.eatright.org

Something Fishy Website on Eating Disorders
www.something-fishy.org

Gurze Books
Tel:(800) 756-7533
www.bulimia.com

If you think that a training partner or friend is struggling with food issues, speak up! Anorexia and bulimia are self-destructive eating behaviors that may signal underlying depression and can be life-threatening. Here are some helpful tips:

- Approach the person gently but be persistent. Say that you are worried about her/his health. S/he, too, may be concerned about her/his loss of concentration, light-headedness, or chronic fatigue. These health changes are more likely to be a stepping stone to accepting help, since the person clings to food and exercise for feelings of control and stability.
- Don't discuss weight or eating habits. Address the fundamental problems of life. Focus on unhappiness as the reason for seeking help. Point out how anxious, tired, and/or irritable the person has been lately. Emphasize that s/he doesn't have to be that way.
- Post a list of resources (with tear-off phone numbers at the bottom) where the person will see it (see resources listed above).

Remember that you are not responsible and can only try to help. Your power comes from using community resources and health professionals, such as a counselor, nutritionist, or eating disorders clinic.

amenorrhea may be an adaptation to the calorie deficit produced either by low calorie intake alone or by increased energy expenditure via exercise. In particular, rapid weight loss may predispose you to amenorrhea. By following a healthy reducing program, such as outlined in Chapter 14, you'll not only have greater success with long-term weight loss, but also have enough energy to run.

3. If you are at an appropriate weight, practice eating as you did as a child: Eat when you are hungry, stop when you are content. If you are always hungry and are constantly obsessing about food, you are undoubtedly trying to eat too few calories. Your body is complaining and requesting more food. Remember that you want to eat adequate calories to support your training program. Chapter 13 can help you determine an appropriate calorie intake and eating schedule that may differ from your current routine, particularly if you yo-yo between starving and bingeing.

4. Eat adequate protein. Research has suggested that amenorrheic runners tend to eat less protein than their regularly menstruating counterparts. In one study, 82 percent of the amenorrheic women ate less than the recommended dietary allowance for protein. Even if you are a vegetarian, remember that you still need adequate protein (see Chapter 5).

5. Eat at least 20 percent of your calories from fat. Amenorrheic marathoners commonly avoid meat and other protein-rich foods because they are afraid of eating fat. They think that if they eat fat, they'll get fat. Although excess calories from fat are easily fattening, some fat (20 to 30 percent of total calories) is an appropriate part of a healthy sports diet. For most active people, this translates into about 40 to 60 or more grams of fat per day. Clearly, this differs from a no-fat diet and allows lean meats, peanut butter, nuts, olive oil, and other wholesome foods that balance a sports diet (see Chapter 6).

6. Include small portions of lean red meat two to four times per week. Surveys of runners show that those with amenorrhea tend to eat less red meat and are more likely to follow a vegetarian diet than their regularly menstruating counterparts. They are also likely to have a diet deficient in iron (see Chapter 5).

Even among nonrunners, vegetarian women are five times more likely to have menstrual problems than meat eaters. It's unclear why meat seems to have a protective effect upon menses. Some researchers believe women who eat meat take in fewer calories from fiber-rich foods. A high-fiber vegetarian diet can alter hormones that affect menses—vegetarians tend to excrete twice as much estrogen as meat eaters. The high fiber intake common to vegetarian diets may also affect calcium absorption, another concern for the amenorrheic woman who needs to optimize calcium intake.

7. *Maintain a calcium-rich diet.* You should choose a high-calcium diet to help maintain bone density. Because you build peak bone density in your teens and early adult years, your goal is to protect against future problems with osteoporosis by eating calcium-rich foods today. As I mentioned in Chapter 1, a safe target is at least 1,000 milligrams of calcium per day if you are between nineteen and fifty years old, and 1,200 to 1,300 milligrams of calcium per day if you are amenorrheic or postmenopausal. This is the equivalent of three to four servings of milk, yogurt, and other dairy or calcium-rich foods per day.

Chapter 1 provides guidelines for getting an optimal amount of calcium. Although you may cringe at the thought of spending so many calories on dairy foods, remember that milk is not an "optional fluid" but rather a wholesome food that contains many important nutrients. Research also suggests women who consume three or more glasses of milk or yogurt per day tend to be leaner than those who do not consume as much dairy. Milk tends to enhance fat loss, not weight gain.

If you are eating a very high-fiber diet (i.e., lots of bran cereal, fruits, and vegetables), you may have a higher need for calcium because the fiber may interfere with calcium absorption. For you, adequate calcium intake will be particularly important.

Calcium is only one factor that affects bone density. Other variables include your genetics, your weight, if and how much you exercise, and how much estrogen you have. There is a genetic factor to osteoporosis; if your mother or grandmother has/had osteoporosis, you are more likely to get the disease. Being too thin, getting inadequate exercise, and having low levels of estrogen also contribute to your risk for osteoporosis. Being athletic, your bones benefit from the protective effect of exercise, particularly strength training, but this does not compensate for being too thin, or having a lack of calcium or a lack of estrogen (as occurs with amenorrhea).

● **SUMMARY**—Food should be one of life's pleasures, a fun part of your marathon training program, and a protector of your good health. If you spend too much time thinking about food as being a fattening enemy, I highly recommend you consult with a registered dietitian who specializes in sports nutrition and eating disorders (use the referral network at www.eatright.org). This professional can help you transform your food fears into healthful fueling, so your body can support your goals of training for and completing the marathon in good health, with high energy.

TRAINING FOR A MARATHON IS A BIG COMMITMENT. IT CONSUMES hours of your time as well as drains both your mental and physical energy. Yet, the process is exciting, rewarding, and hopefully enjoyable. If you are participating in the marathon as a part of a fund raising effort, you gain the additional satisfaction associated with helping to make a difference in the world.

I hope this books helps you enjoy your months of preparation as well as the 26.2 mile event itself. During this process, you'll learn a lot about your body and your stengths, both mental and physical. You'll learn what foods and fluids work and what ones don't. You'll likely be nervous and anxious as the big day draws closer. As one first-time marathoner asked with wringing hands, "Is running a marathon, well... worse than childbirth???" I assured her completing a marathon can be far less painful! It can even be fun.

You've read the tricks on how to keep yourself well fueled and appropriately hydrated. I now wish you the best for your efforts. Have a good one!

—*Nancy Clark*

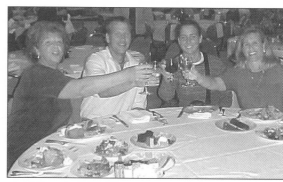

Here's to your good health, high energy and marathon success!

To find a local sports nutritionist contact:

American Dietetic Association
P.O. Box 97215
Chicago, IL 60678
Tel.: (800) 366-1655
Or, use their convenient referral network at *www.eatright.org*

Newsletters

Georgia Tech Sports Medicine & Performance Newsletter
P.O. Box 3000
Denville, NJ 07834
Tel.: (800) 783-4903

Tufts University Health & Nutrition Letter
P.O. Box 420235
Palm Coast, FL 32142-0235
Tel.: (800) 274-7581
http://healthletter.tufts.edu

University of California at Berkeley Wellness Letter
P.O. Box 42018
Palm Coast, FL 32142
Tel.: (386) 447-6328
www.berkeleywellness.com

Catalogs for nutrition books and other resources:

Nutrition topics:
Nutrition Counseling and Education Services
1904 East 123rd Street
Olathe, KS 66061
Tel.: (888) 545-5653
www.ncescatalog.com

Eating disorders:
Gurze Books
P.O. Box 2238
Carlsbad, CA 92018
Tel.: (800) 756-7533
www.bulimia.com

Fitness and sports nutrition:
Human Kinetics
P.O. Box 5076
Champaign, Illinois 61825-5076
Tel.: (800) 747-4457
www.humankinetics.com

Recommended Books:

Benardot, Dan. *Nutrition for Serious Athletes.* Human Kinetics, 2000.

Clark, Nancy. *Nancy Clark's Sports Nutrition Guidebook, Second Edition.* Human Kinetics, 1997.

Dorfman, Lisa. *The Vegetarian Sports Nutrition Guide: Peak Performance for Everyone from Beginners to Gold Medalists.* John Wiley & Sons, Inc., 1999.

Duyff, Roberta. *The American Dietetic Association's Complete Food and Nutrition Guide.* Chronimed Publishing, 1998.

Hall, Lindsey. *Full Lives: Women Who Have Freed Themselves from Food & Weight Obsession.* Gurze Books, 1993.

Hirschmann, Jane and Carol Munter. *When Women Stop Hating Their Bodies: Freeing Yourself from Food and Weight Obsession.* Fawcett Books, 1997.

LoBue, Andrea & Marsea Marcus. *The Don't Diet, Live-It! Workbook: Healing Food, Weight & Body Issues.* Gurze Books, 1999.

Satter, Ellyn. *Secrets of Feeding a Healthy Family.* Kelcy Press, 1999.

Michelle, Judith Brisman, and Margot Weinshel. *Surviving an Eating Disorder: Strategies for Families and Friends.* HarperCollins, 1997.

Tribole, Evelyn and Elyse Resch. *Intuitive Eating: A Recovery Book for the Chronic Dieter: Rediscover the Pleasures of Eating and Rebuild Your Body Image.* St Martins Mass Market, 1996.

For coaches and professionals:

Rosenbloom, Christine. *Sports Nutrition: A Guide for the Professional Working with Active People*, third edition. American Dietetics Association, 2000.

Internet Resources

Sports and sports nutrition:

Nancy Clark, MS, RD
www.nancyclarkrd.com
> Links to nutrition articles and other nutrition sources; information on teaching materials

Australian Institute of Sport
www.ais.org.au/nutrition
> Comprehensive information on physical fitness and nutrition

Gatorade Sports Science Institute
www.gssiweb.com
> Information on endurance sports nutrition

Sportscience
www.sportsci.org
> An interdisciplinary site for research on human physical performance

WaddleOn.com
www.waddleon.com
> An Internet guide to becoming an athlete, whatever your size or shape

Health and nutrition:

ConsumerLab.com
www.consumerlab.com
> Independently tests nutritional supplements and posts the results.

International Food Information Council Foundation
http://ific.org
> Geared mostly to health professionals, the site features information on food safety and nutrition.

National Library of Medicine, U.S. Department of Health and Human Services
www.nlm.nih.gov
> Free access to medical journals

U.S. Department of Health and Human Services
www.healthfinder.gov
> Provides information and lists publications and not-for-profit organizations that produce reliable information.

Eating disorders:

National Eating Disorders Association
www.NationalEatingDisorders.org
> Information, resources, and links for eating disorders

Something Fishy Website on Eating Disorders
www.something-fishy.org
> Offers extensive resources and referrals for eating disorders.

SELECTED REFERENCES

American Dietetic Association, American College of Sports Medicine, and Dietitians of Canada. "Joint Position Statement: Nutrition and Athletic Performance." *Journal of the American Dietetic Association* 12 (2000): 1543–56.

Beals, K. and M. Manore. "Behavioral, Psychological, and Physical Characteristics of Female Athletes with Subclinical Eating Disorders." *International Journal of Sports Nutrition and Exercise Metabolism* 10, no. 2 (2000): 128–43.

Brouns, F., W. Saris, and N. Rehrer. "Abdominal Complaints and Gastro-Intestinal Function During Long-Lasting Exercise." *International Journal of Sports Medicine* 8 (1987): 175–89.

Bouchard, C., et al. "The Response to Long Term Overfeeding in Identical Twins." *New England Journal of Medicine* 322 (1990): 1477–82.

Burke, L. "Nutritional Needs for Exercise in the Heat." *Comparative Biochemistry and Physiology A—Mol Integr Physiol* 128, no. 4 (2001): 735–48.

Burke, L., G. Collier, and M. Hargreaves. "Glycemic Index—a New Tool in Sport Nutrition?" *International Journal of Sports Nutrition* 8 (1998): 401–15.

Carrithers, J.A., et al. "Effects of Post-Exercise Protein-Carbohydrate Feedings on Muscle Glycogen Restoration." *Journal of Applied Physiology* 88, no. 6 (2000): 1976–82.

Casa, D., et al. "National Athletic Trainers' Association Position Statement: Fluid Replacement for Athletes." *Journal of Athletic Training* 35, no. 2 (2000): 212–24.

Clark, N., M. Nelson, and W. Evans. "Nutrition Education for Elite Women Runners." *Physician and Sportsmedicine* 16, no. 2 (1988): 124–34.

Garner, D. "The Effects of Starvation on Behavior: Implications for Dieting and Eating Disorders." *Healthy Weight Journal* 12, no. 5 (1998): 68–72.

Hagberg, J., et al. "Determinants of Body Composition in Post-Menopausal Women." *Journal of Gerontology A—Biol Sci Med Sci* 55, no. 10 (2000): M607–12.

Hill, R.J. and P.S. Davies. "The Validity of Self-Reported Energy Intake as Determined Using the Doubly Labeled Water Technique." *British Journal of Nutrition* 85, no. 4 (2001): 415–30.

Jakicic, J., et al. "American College of Sports Medicine Position Stand. Appropriate Intervention Strategies for Weight Loss and Prevention of Weight Regain for Adults." *Medicine and Science in Sports and Exercise* 12 (2001): 2145–56.

Malcsewska, J., G. Raczynski, and R. Stupnicki. "Iron Status in Female Endurance Athletes and Non-Athletes." *International Journal of Sports Nutrition and Exercise Metabolism* 10, no. 3 (2000): 260–76.

Nativ, A. "Stress Fractures and Bone Health in Track and Field Athletes." *Journal of Science and Medicine in Sport* 3, no. 3 (2000): 268–79.

Neiman, D. "Physical Fitness and Vegetarian Diets: Is There a Relation?" *American Journal of Clinical Nutrition* 70, no. 3 Suppl. (1999): 570S–75S.

Pedersen, A., et al. "Menstrual Differences Due to Vegetarian and Non-Vegetarian Diets." *American Journal of Clinical Nutrition* 53 (1991): 879–85.

Pendergast, D., J. Leddy, and J. Veentkatraman. "A Perspective on Fat Intake in Athletes." *Journal of the American College of Nutrition* 19, no. 3 (2000): 345–50.

Rehrer, N. "Fluid and Electrolyte Balance in Ultra-Endurance Sport." *Sports Medicine* 31, no. 10 (2001): 701–15.

Sanborn, C.F., B. Albrecht, and W. Wagner. "Athletic Amenorrhea: Lack of Association with Body Fat." *Medicine and Science in Sports and Exercise* 19, no. 3 (1987): 207–12.

Sanborn, C.F., et al. "Disordered Eating and the Female Athlete Triad." *Clinical Sports Medicine* 19, no. 2 (2000): 199–213.

Schulz, L.O., et al. "Energy Expenditure of Elite Female Runners Measured by Respiratory Chamber and Doubly Labeled Water." *Journal of Applied Physiology* 72, no. 1 (1992): 23–28.

Sherman, W.M. "Muscle Glycogen Supercompensation During the Week Before Athletic Competition." *Sports Science Exchange* (The Gatorade Institute) 2, no. 16 (1989).

Wilmore, J., et al. "Is There Energy Conservation in Amenorrheic Compared with Eumenorrheic Distance Runners?" *Journal of Applied Physiology* 72, no. 1 (1992): 15–22.

Zelasko, C. "Exercise for Weight Loss: What Are the Facts?" *Journal of the American Dietetic Association* 95 (1995): 1414–17.

Alcoholic beverages:
  diuretic effect of, 94
  fluid replacement with, 63
  as recovery fluid, 85
Amenorrhea:
  causes of, 125, 129
  definition of, 125
  and health risks, 126
  resolving, 126, 127-130
  risk factors for, 125
  and a vegetarian diet, 130
American College of Sports Medicine, 58
American Dietetic Association, 123, 128
  See also Dietitians
American Heart Association, 45
Amino Acids. *See* Protein
Anemia, iron-deficiency:
  and fatigue, 36
  prevention of, 16, 40
  See also Iron
Animal fats. *See* Fats, dietary
Anorexia. *See* Eating disorders
Antioxidants. *See* Vitamins, anti-oxidant
Appetite:
  controlling, 8, 17, 18, 24, 31, 32, 104
  morning, 17
  natural, 104
  post-exercise, 81
  on weight reduction diet, 105, 109,
    113, 114
Ascorbic acid. *See* Vitamin C
Balanced diet, 4
Banana Bread, 20 (recipe)
Bananas:
  carbohydrate in, 83 (table)
  recipes with:
    Banana Bread, 20
Bean Dip, 50 (recipe)
Beans, dried (legumes):
  health benefits of, 36, 44
  as iron source, 46 (table)
  as protein source, 42 (table), 43
  serving suggestions for, 25 (table), 44
  recipes with:
    Bean Dip, 50
    Chicken and Black Bean Soup, 86
Beans and rice. *See* Protein, combining
Beef. *See* Meat
Beer, 59 (table)
  See also alcoholic beverages
Beta carotene, 5
  See also Vitamins, anti-oxidant

Beverages:
  pre-exercise, 71
  See also Alcoholic beverages; Fluids;
Water
  recipes for:
    Homemade Sports Drink, 64
Blood glucose. *See* Blood sugar
Blood pressure. *See* High blood pressure
Blood sugar:
  low (hypoglycemia), 37, 70, 73
  maintaining normal level during
    exercise, 68, 75, 77
  See also Glycemic index
Body fat:
  and amenorrhea, 125
  burning versus losing, 111
  essential, 123
  gender differences in, 116, 122, 123
  variability in
Body image, 116, 123
Bone density, 7, 126, 130
Bones:
  and osteoporosis, 126
  stress fractures, 47, 126
Bonking. See "Hitting the wall"
Bowel movements. *See* Constipation;
    Diarrhea; Fiber; Digestion; Stomach
Bran cereals, 16
  See also Fiber
Breads:
  as protein source 42 (table)
  See also Carbohydrates; Grains
    and starches
  recipe for: Banana Bread, 20
Breakfast:
  balanced, 19
  digesting, 16
  as dining-out meal, 98
  for early-morning exercisers, 15
  as most important meal of day, 14
  non-traditional, 15
  pre-event, 94
  recipes for, 20
  as recovery meal, 16
  skipping, 14, 111
  suggestions for, 14, 15, 41, 98
  See also Breads; Breakfast cereals
Breakfast cereals:
  choosing, 16, 17
  fat in, 17
  fiber-rich, 16
  as protein source, 42 (table)

Nancy Clark, M.S., R.D., an internationally known sports nutritionist, is Director of Nutrition Services for SportsMedicine Associates, one of the largest athletic injury clinics in New England. A registered dietitian specializing in nutrition for exercise, wellness, and the management of eating disorders, Clark counsels both casual exercisers and competitive athletes at her Boston-area office. Her more famous clients include members of the Boston Red Sox, Boston Celtics and many elite and Olympic athletes. She is the nutrition consultant to Boston College's Sports Medicine Department and the Arthritis Foundation's Joints in Motion national marathon training program.

Clark is the author of the best-seller *Nancy Clark's Sports Nutrition Guidebook* (Human Kinetics; first edition,1990; second edition 1997), a book commonly referred to as the "sports nutrition bible." A regular contributor to *SHAPE* and *Runner's World* magazines, Clark also writes a monthly nutrition column called "The Athlete's Kitchen" which appears regularly in over 100 sports and health publications, including *New England Runner*. She is also author of *The New York City Marathon Cookbook*.

Clark completed her undergraduate degree in nutrition from Simmons College in Boston, her dietetic internship at Massachusetts General Hospital, and her graduate degree in nutrition with a focus on exercise physiology from Boston University. She is a Fellow of both the American Dietetic Association and the American College of Sports Medicine and is a member of the Sports Medicine Referral Network for USA Gymnastics and USA Swimming.

Sports and nutrition are personal as well as professional interests for Clark. As a member of the Greater Boston Track Club, she has competed at the 10-kilometer, half-marathon, and marathon distances and was instrumental in founding the Boston Milk Run, a nationally recognized road race sponsored by the Massachusetts Dietetic Association. An avid bike-commuter, Clark has led extended bike tours, including Bikecentennial's Trans-America Trip and tours through the Canadian and Colorado Rockies. She has trekked in the Himalayas and helped to plan a menu for a successful mountain climbing expedition. She lives with her husband, son, and daughter in Newton, MA.

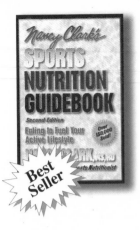

"Nancy Clark's Sports Nutrition Guidebook *is my nutrition bible. It helped me lose weight, improve my eating, boost my energy, and feel stronger."*

If you like *Nancy Clark's Food Guide for Marathoners*, you'll also like *Nancy Clark's Sports Nutrition Guidebook*. With more than 250,000 copies in print, this best seller is a comprehensive resource. The 456 fact-filled pages are divided into four sections:
• daily eating on the run
• sports nutrition for both casual and competitive athletes
• weight management issues and eating disorders
• quick and easy recipes that support healthful eating.

"Clark's tape on Dieting Tips for Active People *is actually helpful. I've lost three pounds already and feel more at peace with food."*

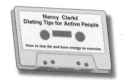

Clark's 40 minute tape can help you have energy to enjoy exercising even when you are losing body fat.

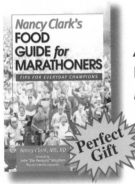

Are your peers struggling with low energy? **Nancy Clark's Food Guide for Marathoners** *makes the perfect gift.*

ORDER FORM: ▬ ▬ ▬ ▬ ▬ ▬ ▬ ▬ ▬ ▬ ▬ ▬ ▬ ▬ ▬ ▬ ▬

☐ Sports Nutrition Guidebook, $19
☐ Food Guide for Marathoners, $15
☐ Weight loss audiotape, $10
Postage + $5, $2 every additional item; Mass. residents add 5% sales tax.

Name:_____
Address: _____
City, State, Zip: _____
Phone: _____
email: _____

Enclosed is a check payable to :

Sports Nutrition Publishers
60 Lindbergh Ave Suite 3A
West Newton, MA 02465
www.nancyclarkrd.com
Phone: 617-795-0823; Fax: 617-795-1876

Please charge to: ☐ Visa ☐ Mastercard

Card number: _____
Exp. Date: _____
Signature:_____

☐ *I'd like more information about Clark's nutrition education materials: handouts and powerpoint presentations on sports nutrition and weight management*